'Nicola's approach t~~...~~
and insightful, this boo~~k is a bible~~
with lots of great advice'
ALESHA DiXON

'This book will supercharge your wellbeing practices.
A fresh, personalized toolkit, tailored to your needs,
your preferences and your available resources'
SUZY READING,
Chartered Psychologist

'An invaluable guide to holistic wellbeing.
This book holds a permanent spot on the shelf
in my therapy practice'
JOSHUA FLETCHER
(@anxietyjosh) Anxiety therapist and author

'This book has the power to relax you,
pick you up when you need it or make you
feel comforted in times of need'
BRYONY BLAKE,
Celebrity make-up artist

THE FOUR WAYS TO WELLBEING

Nicola Elliott is the Founder and Creative Director of NEOM, the award-winning wellbeing brand. She worked for ten years as a journalist in London, on magazines including *Glamour*, *InStyle* and *Marie Claire*, and decided to launch NEOM after experimenting with essential oil blends and discovering the power they hold to tackle the stress and demands of modern-day life. The company that started with a few blends created for family and friends has now grown into a brand present in over 500 stores across the UK and worldwide. This is her first book.

THE FOUR WAYS TO WELLBEING

Better Sleep. Less Stress.
More Energy. Mood Boost.

NICOLA ELLIOTT, FOUNDER OF NEOM

PENGUIN LIFE

AN IMPRINT OF

PENGUIN BOOKS

PENGUIN LIFE

UK | USA | Canada | Ireland | Australia
India | New Zealand | South Africa

Penguin Life is part of the Penguin Random House group of companies
whose addresses can be found at global.penguinrandomhouse.com.

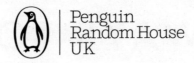

First published 2024
001

Copyright © Nicola Elliott, 2024

The moral right of the author has been asserted

Set in 9.5/14.75pt Museo Slab Std
Typeset by Jouve (UK), Milton Keynes
Printed and bound in Great Britain by Clays Ltd, Elcograf S.p.A.

The authorized representative in the EEA is Penguin Random House Ireland,
Morrison Chambers, 32 Nassau Street, Dublin D02 YH68

A CIP catalogue record for this book is available from the British Library

ISBN: 978-0-241-66006-5

www.greenpenguin.co.uk

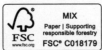

Penguin Random House is committed to a
sustainable future for our business, our readers
and our planet. This book is made from Forest
Stewardship Council® certified paper.

Charlie and Alexa. Always remember the three things: be kind, work hard, have fun xxx

CONTENTS

Foreword   ix

INTRODUCTION   1
   Welcome to the world of NEOM   3
   NEOM's manifesto   4
   So, let's talk about wellbeing . . .   5
   The four ways to wellbeing   9
   How it all began and the story of NEOM   15
   The natural power of essential oils   22
   My am to pm NEOM wellbeing wonders   32
   It's just my opinion, but . . .   33
   Tips on how to use this book   37
1. SLEEP   41
2. STRESS   111
3. ENERGY   159
4. MOOD   203

Conclusion   239
Nicola's Little Black Book of Wellbeing   241
Notes   257

FOREWORD

Hello, I'm Nicola and founder of NEOM.

Whatever your mind and body needs, I'm here to help you master the four ways to better wellbeing. I've done all the work so you don't have to and have compiled the very best of what I've learned, in over eighteen years of building an award-winning wellbeing brand. I've been there, tried that and got the weighted blanket; I know what works and what doesn't, whose advice to listen to and why balance is more about enjoying that glass of wine than holding a tree pose! So whether you've got 5 minutes to dip in with your morning coffee, or 30 minutes to read in the bathtub, here's your chance to access my top picks of the industry's finest real-world tips, tricks and exercises. With something to suit everyone from green goddesses to the totally overwhelmed, now's the opportunity to arm yourself with the small steps, practices and knowledge to help you on your own journey to better sleep, less stress, more energy and a lifted mood. Enjoy the ride.

Nicola

Nicola x
@nicolaelliottneom

INTRODUCTION

WELCOME TO THE WORLD OF NEOM

* Founded in 2005
* 100% natural fragrances used in every product
* One candle sold every 45 seconds*
* One Perfect Night's Pillow Mist sold every 3 minutes*
* Certified B Corporation since 2022
* Proud to partner with the Mental Health Foundation charity since 2020

Global sales data at time of going to print

NEOM'S MANIFESTO

At NEOM, we believe wellbeing starts with the little moments . . .

The deeply relaxing bath that prepares you for *better sleep*. The candle that creates a calm zone and *less stress* in your busy family home. The shower wash that helps you have *more energy* and ready to kick ass at 6am. The hand balm in your bag with the power to help give you a daily *mood boost*.

Our fragrances are 100% *natural* with true wellbeing benefits: to help you sleep better, stress less, boost your energy or lift your mood.

Our mission is to *supercharge* wellbeing . . . not only of our communities but for our planet too. We want to leave both in a better place.

All our products are made with botanical ingredients and 100% naturally derived wax, and we use 100% natural fragrances to boost your wellbeing.

SO, LET'S TALK
ABOUT WELLBEING . . .

'Wellbeing isn't about being super virtuous and not having any fun.'

Wellbeing is a massive topic these days. I love that, because it means we're thinking and talking about it. The downside is a lot of us don't really know *what* it means and *where* to start. When I started NEOM, my mantra was 'small steps, big difference'. Just like anything, the journey of a thousand miles starts with taking that first step.

After nearly two decades working in the wellness industry, I've heard thousands of customer stories, as well as being in the privileged position of having access to the best experts, which is why I'm super excited to bring you this book. With everything I have learned and the best advice I have gathered about wellbeing distilled down into one easy, achievable guide, you'll come away being able to devise your own personalized toolkit.

I'm passionate about wellbeing but I've always had a No BS approach to knowing the difference between what is a fad and what actually works. Right from the get-go at NEOM we've been fanatical about making sure everything is evidence-based and from experts and professionals, which is what you'll find here in this book.

I'm still on my own wellbeing journey myself, because like all of us, my needs change every year – and sometimes every week! I'm always looking for new ways to improve my sleep, stress, energy and mood and I like to keep it pretty simple. If you're sleeping the best you can, and you've got your stress in check, you can make a material impact on your energy levels, and therefore your mood is also something you have control and balance over. That's both a reassuring and really empowering place to start.

YOU are the most important project you'll **EVER** work on

YOU DO YOU

There's a myth around wellbeing that you have to do things a certain way, but the reality is that everyone's needs are different. One thing we're clear on at NEOM is that wellbeing is a very personal thing. One person may need to sleep for 7 hours, another for 10. Someone else could love doing HIIT classes, while another person likes walking in nature, while for someone else it's a Joe Wicks workout in the kitchen after dropping the kids off at school. Some people like to meditate in a certain way, while others might get their calm with a 10-minute soak in the bath, or curling up with a good book.

Whatever it looks like to you, it should feel good. Wellbeing is something that we should enjoy and celebrate. There's often the disconnect in which people assume it's about either leading a 'naughty' but fun life, or a 'good' life that's super virtuous and – well – a bit boring. I've never been someone who's got up at 6am to make a green smoothie and do yoga on the beach. That's just not what wellbeing looks like to me. I don't like running or the taste of matcha tea, and I prefer milk chocolate to dark. You've got to find what's right – and most importantly what's enjoyable – for you.

There's no
right or wrong
way to do
WELLBEING

What works for me is sticking to a sleep routine and the mood boost I get after exercising for 30 minutes. I also definitely notice the difference in my energy levels when I'm eating more wholefoods as opposed to processed stuff. But absolutely under no circumstance would I ever forgo a decent bottle of white wine. Wellbeing is something that should be nice, nourishing and makes you feel good. It's all about balance and being forgiving to yourself when sometimes things go a bit awry.

SMALL STEPS

It's also important to say that your wellbeing isn't a predetermined state. It's not that you either sleep well or don't sleep well, or that you're a stressed person or a not stressed person. You have material control over those areas in your life. Wellbeing starts with the right mindset. Our philosophy at NEOM has always been 'small steps, big difference' for a reason. If there's any secret to wellbeing, this is it: small things done on a consistent basis can ladder up to have a hugely positive effect.

DEMYSTIFYING WELLBEING

There can be a lot of alchemy and hype around wellbeing, as if it's something complicated or mysterious that only a few enlightened people know about. My mission is to democratize wellbeing and make it available for all. This book recognizes the reality of your busy lifestyle, but it also gives you the tools and knowledge to empower yourself. If you're willing to start your journey, take some small steps every day with enthusiasm to experiment and find out what your own wellbeing toolkit is, then you've reached what we call utopia at NEOM. No matter how it might feel sometimes, you're in control of your own destiny, and that's what is really exciting.

Ready to take that first (small) step?

Small steps BIG difference

THE FOUR WAYS TO WELLBEING

Before we dive in, let's have a look at the fundamentals. I always think of wellbeing within the context of our four pillars: better sleep, less stress, more energy and boosting mood. Everything we create at NEOM sits within one of those, and everything in this book does too.

SLEEP

'The power to better sleep is in our hands.'

To me, sleep is the bedrock of better wellbeing. I think you never look or feel your best without a good night's sleep, and it's the absolute foundation for being able to deal with stress, regulate mood, boost energy and everything else in between.

At the other end of the scale, too little sleep has been linked to a host of wider issues, from weakened immunity and digestive systems to memory and mental health. Obviously, we won't sleep brilliantly all the time and we're not going to fall into a pit after the odd night or even a week of bad sleep, but the importance of sleep is unarguable. Yet it's often the first thing to slip down the list of our priorities as our busy lives fill up with commitments that leave us little time to get into a healthy, sufficient routine that works for us. We end up fitting sleep in around our life, which can actually have a really detrimental effect on the life we live.

We have been on the NEOM sleep journey for almost twenty years – from researching techniques to creating products that help people all over the world get a perfect night's sleep – and the great thing that we've learned is that we don't have to stay stuck in the cycle; we really can take steps and influence how well we sleep. The power is in our hands. It's not a case of 'I'm a good sleeper or a bad sleeper,' or 'My mum/gran/great-uncle Norman was an insomniac, it runs in the family.' There are material things you can do to change how you sleep. In Chapter 1 you're going to discover the 11 Golden Rules for Better Sleep, where we put together the most fascinating, game-changing tips in one achievable plan. I can't tell you the difference it made to my sleep after only a few days. The 11 Golden Rules revolutionize the way we should be looking at sleep, and in particular the role light plays in it. This first chapter unpicks all the common sleep myths and gives you all the little tips and tricks to optimize your sleep. Get this pillar right and there's a pretty good chance that the others will follow.

STRESS

'Stress is a marker to tell us when things are getting too much.'

Although it might feel like a modern problem that has taken over since the dawn of emails and traffic jams, stress is hardwired into us and is actually very normal and healthy in the right amounts. If you're reading this and feel that your stress is spiralling out of control, that it's threatening to overwhelm you, or it's got to the point that it's having a detrimental impact on your health and your life, it's really important that you reach out to the right people and/or a trusted health professional. But when I talk about stress here, it's in the context of reframing it as something that is normal, manageable and, well, something not to get too stressed about.

Stress is vital for two important functions. The first is our fight or flight mode, which is the innate response our body goes into when it senses danger, as a biological mechanism designed to keep us safe. Our heart rate and blood pressure rise and our senses become sharper, meaning we become faster, stronger and more alert. We might not be running away from the hungry lion or facing life-and-death situations like our ancestors once were, but today we're facing a different set of problems. Trying to find a decent work–life balance, making enough money to look after our families, dealing with health worries or just trying to manage the daily juggle can all fill up our stress bucket and the cumulative effect is that we feel constantly on edge.

Stress can also be a productive and motivating force. Studies from the University of California, Berkeley, have found that moderate, short-lived stress can improve alertness and performance and boost memory. In the right context a little bit of stress can be a good thing and we shouldn't be scared of it. It's just about keeping things in check and, as you'll see, it's perfectly possible to do that.

The other great thing is that reducing our stress levels can have an upstream effect. If we're better equipped to teach ourselves how to deal with difficult situations, it can help us lead a fuller, more balanced life. If we learn how to manage our stress, we can take on bigger things, like projects or life decisions that might have felt too scary or overwhelming in the past. It's not just the health benefits of reducing stress: it's about getting our armour in place so we can go and live our best, biggest and most adventurous life. To me, that's a really important part of the 'why' around learning these wellbeing tools.

ENERGY

'A lack of energy is one of the biggest reasons for opting out of life.'

Energy and sleep are probably the two pillars most closely tied to each other. It goes without saying that getting too little sleep will affect your energy, and vice versa. From all the thousands of people I've interacted with over the years, I've seen first hand how having little or no energy is one of the main reasons people don't get involved in things and opt out of the good bits of life, whether that be going to a really fun party or social gathering, taking up something new or pushing yourself out of your comfort zone at work. If you haven't got any energy, you haven't got the motivation or joy to take part. Again, that seems like a really fixable reason to start showing up for yourself by taking simple steps to improve your wellbeing.

One of the problems is that energy can be a bit of a chicken and egg scenario. Studies from Harvard Medical School have proven that exercise boosts energy levels, but it can be near impossible if you've got no get-up-and-go in the first place. We've had people come into our NEOM Wellbeing Hubs and one of the main reasons they're not exercising is because they've got no energy, which in turn gives them even less energy, and that can become a vicious circle.

Even if we do exercise or consider ourselves to be an active person, we might be doing less than we think. A recent study from University College London showed that 74 per cent of British middle-aged adults spend more than 8 hours sitting each day. Unsurprisingly for those in their forties, a quarter of this time is made up of prolonged bouts of sitting for an hour or more at a time. An overbusy mind combined with an underbusy body is something most of us can probably identify with. If you're suffering from extreme exhaustion or persistent fatigue it's advisable to get checked out by your GP, but feeling generally tired or subpar most of the time doesn't have to be something we just accept as part of life's deal. By implementing small tweaks we can tangibly lift our energy levels and fire up our day, and that knowledge alone gives me life – I hope it does for you, too.

MOOD

'You can't stop the waves but you can learn to surf.'

– Jon Kabat-Zinn

Mood is the hardest pillar to define but what we all want is to feel happy, right? But happiness is subjective and can mean different things to everyone. For me, it's sunny mornings and going horse riding with my daughter, but for others it might be gardening, cooking, or even something as simple as having an empty laundry basket or fresh sheets on the bed (I know people for whom that is their idea of heaven).

Whatever our version of happiness is, having a balanced mood and a more positive state of mind is a really great starting point. Like stress, it might sometimes seem like our mood is completely out of our control, but I'm pleased to say that there are things we can do to make sure our mood doesn't drastically swing up and down too much. If we can create that pendulum of balance, we're going to have the foundation for living our best life.

Over the last four decades our views on our mood and minds have changed significantly, with the knowledge that we have more control of our mindset than previously thought. Today it's generally accepted that the adult brain is far from being 'fixed'. In recent years there's been a huge amount of research into neuroplasticity, which is the brain's ability to rewire, relearn and strengthen important neural connections, enabling us to think and respond differently to things. We'll be delving deeper into neuroplasticity on page 211, but the science now shows that we literally have the ability to change the way we think, and how we see ourselves and interact with the world.

HOW IT ALL BEGAN
AND THE STORY OF NEOM

My own wellbeing journey arose out of a moment in time – when life was, shall we say, particularly hectic. It was 2005 and I was living in London and working as an editor for a glossy lifestyle magazine. I was out at launches and parties most nights and flying all over the world interviewing celebrities, but I was also working 60 hours a week with constant deadlines and in a culture that meant you were never 'off'.

Despite having what I considered my dream job, plus a really fun social life, I started having panic attacks. I would start sweating and having out-of-body experiences at the most random and mundane moments, like when I was at home, or in a meeting, or sitting on the bus on the way into work. It felt really scary at the time because I'd always been a pretty healthy and grounded person and I didn't know what was happening to me.

Looking back, I was just squeezing too much stuff in. I think it's important to recognize that. It's not always when you've gone through a really turbulent time, or something huge has happened that anxiety arises. Even when things are fine, or even going really well, we can put ourselves under too much pressure. It's not possible to run on empty so we have to stop and replenish the cup sometimes.

HOME TRUTHS

One evening, in the midst of this hectic era, I remember ringing my mum because I had got to a point where I knew I needed some advice. She told me: 'You're just not looking after yourself. It's as simple as that.' The difference was, back then, in 2005, the word 'wellbeing' didn't exist. People didn't really go to gyms or think about their sleep or energy levels or mood states. It just wasn't a *thing*. I'll admit that I knew very little about diet, nutrition or the importance of movement beyond looking good! I was twenty-two and living on very little sleep and pesto pasta, because I thought that was the healthy option. I wasn't getting up before midday on a weekend and I was working all week until late, not taking lunch hours, partying all week and not prioritizing sleep. The basic boxes weren't being ticked. It's hardly surprising that when I started having panic attacks, my mum told me in her very no-nonsense northern tone: 'You've got to look after yourself. The basics are really important. Start eating proper meals, get outdoors and see the sunshine, take it easy and calm down.'

At the top of my road where I lived there was what I'd call a typical nineties health food shop. It had a sorry-looking fruit bowl in the window with a solitary banana and everything inside was a bit dusty and uninspiring. There were none of the lovely health food stores you get now, like Fresh & Wild and Planet Organic. But this shop did have a small range of essential oils, which even though I hadn't really thought much of or even tried before, really interested me; not only did they smell really lovely, they also had some information that talked about how they could help you feel better. And I thought, wouldn't it be great to be able to create little natural potions of my own that could help, dependent on how I was feeling.

THE FOUR PILLARS

I started making my own blends, from refreshing oils that helped enliven me and lavender oils that helped me relax, and I really started to see and feel a difference. Before long, my friends and family were asking me to start making them blends as well. It soon became clear that everyone around me seemed to suffer from four things: poor sleep, lack of energy, mood imbalance or stress. That's where I came up with the concept of the four pillars, or 'modern malaises' as I call them, which became the foundations of NEOM. And, more than likely, one of these things would lead to another. So if you've got one issue, you've probably got two. That's the thing about wellbeing; it's like an ecosystem and not something that works independently of anything else. When one goes down, there's a pretty good chance they're all going to follow.

At the time my sister worked for Friends of the Earth and would only use natural-based products, whereas I worked in magazines where we discussed all the latest products in the beauty world, and none were natural then. Naturally derived beauty products that were made without synthetic ingredients weren't really on anyone's radar, but I was intrigued by the power of using ingredients and essential oils that had been used for their therapeutic benefits for such a long time. When it came to setting up NEOM, I knew we had to use essential oils, because they were the things that were really going to move the dial and make the difference to help people with their wellbeing.

WELLBEING FOR MODERN LIFE

I was learning fast that all aspects of wellbeing had to work hand in hand. I wanted to learn more about essential oils, so I did a learn-at-home aromatherapy course alongside training as a nutritionist. That gave me the basic theory I needed but for the practical elements I was mostly learning on the job. I was soon busy experimenting with different blends such as lemon and peppermint, which are known for their stimulating and invigorating properties and focusing the mind.

My boyfriend at the time used to come back from playing football on a Saturday and have no energy to go out that night, so I created an oil with a real energy-boosting fragrance that included lemon and basil essential oils to put in his bath and it really helped him. It's a blend we have still at NEOM today, and is called Feel Refreshed. I remember thinking at the time that these were very real-life issues that people were experiencing but the only blends I could find were labelled vague things like 'inspiration' and 'joy'. I thought, what does that actually mean? There was no one doing blends that would truly help me or the people I knew. The amazing power of these essential oils just hadn't been reimagined for modern life – and that's where my idea for NEOM was born.

From conception to launching NEOM took a year. I initially went down to working four days a week at the magazine and then worked Fridays, Saturdays and Sundays on the business. I can't deny, there was some juggling of taking phone calls in the toilets at work; I then managed to negotiate going down to three days a week. I sold my car to raise money and used the spare room in my flat as a little stockroom. After a year, when I started getting enough interest from independent stockists, it felt like enough of a green light to hand in my notice and go full-time with the business. One thing I get asked quite a bit is how to start a business and I always say: start it as a side hustle or treat it as a hobby you have enough interest in that you want to keep going. You don't have to go all in and chuck in the day job right at the start; financially that wasn't viable for me at the time anyway. We originally launched with four candles based around our well-being pillars and over the years have branched out into products for the bath, body and skin.

The turning point was going to a trade show and explaining to people that at the time, the majority of candles weren't made of naturally derived waxes or natural fragrances. People were lighting candles because they wanted some sort of benefit for themselves, so offering a natural alternative really engaged them and felt like a real light-bulb moment. I remember looking at the long queue of people at our stand wanting to know more and realizing that was a really good sign. At the start those four candles included our Feel Refreshed fragrance and our Perfect Night's Sleep fragrance with up to nineteen essential oils including lavender, which I'd created for my sister when she had trouble sleeping. That's where we were (and always have been) really different at NEOM. We look at what is happening in the real world and create products to solve that problem: the person who is feeling stressed, or who hasn't had a good night's sleep, or needs a boost going into a morning meeting. Real modern-life situations where natural solutions can help make all the difference.

'We had the amazing power of these essential oils but they hadn't been reimagined for modern life.'

Nearly two decades on, we still start all our product development in that way. We think 'what are people going through right now?'

or maybe collectively we're feeling a bit down about what's happening in the world, or we need to create an inspiring, energizing space to work from home, or it might be someone studying or sitting their university exams and needing to switch their brain on.

ANCIENT INSPIRATION

What's crazy is that this is actually ancient technology that we have lost touch with over the last few centuries. Plant extracts have been used for their health properties for thousands of years to treat everything from pain relief, digestion and skin problems to sleep and nerve disorders – two thousand years ago the Romans were using lavender in their baths to relax and soothe themselves, as we still do today. Modern research has shown that elements of these ingredients can interact with the limbic part of the brain, which controls things like heart rate, blood pressure, hormone balance, as well as emotional and behavioural responses. When we know how to harness them, we can use them in specific ways to make a real impact on how we feel in terms of our sleep, stress, energy and mood state. I'll be delving further into how essential oils work on page 22; it's a truly fascinating process.

KNOW YOUR NEEDS

When it comes to wellbeing, our needs change throughout our lives. Obviously my needs as a 44-year-old mum of two are very different to that 22-year-old party-going woman, just as my wellbeing needs change from summer to winter. For women especially, it's multifaceted. It can depend on where we are in our hormone cycle, and whether we're starting our periods or going through the menopause. It depends on what's going on in our lives. Are we stressed? Happy? Taking on too much? Maybe we've just found out we're pregnant with our first child, or we're going through a divorce or have suffered a bereavement. People have very different needs at different times and that's why their wellbeing toolkit will look different. My own experience of anxiety and burnout taught me that our wellbeing is impacted by whatever is going on in our lives, and that sometimes we need to stop, take a step back and think about what we need.

YOUR BEST IS ENOUGH

To me, wellbeing has always been about feeling our personal best. It's about being aware of all the ways we can feed our bodies and minds, so we physically and mentally squeeze the best out of life. I won't pretend I always get it right because my halo slips rather often, but that's all part of the fun and just being, well, human.

One of the questions I get asked is how I manage to run a business alongside having a family, as well as making time for myself. My answer to that is simple: you have to get comfortable dropping balls. You can't always do it all the way you'd like to. It's about sometimes making decisions where you're 51 per cent happy with something, because done is better than perfect. There's not a magic formula. It's not by working harder or staying up later. It's just doing your best, getting it wrong occasionally and being OK with that. So as my mum would say, look after yourself, take accountability where you can, enjoy the process and, most importantly, cut yourself some slack sometimes. That's the definition of true wellbeing and a life lived well.

THE NATURAL POWER
OF ESSENTIAL OILS

As I talked about earlier, my essential oil journey started from humble beginnings back in 2005 when I was suffering with burnout. I stumbled across what felt like these undiscovered, miraculous ingredients in my local dusty health shop and became interested in the concept of being able to do something to affect yourself positively without taking a pill, in the more pleasant and nurturing environment of your own home.

Aromatherapy is the practice of using essential oils for their aromatherapeutic benefits. The first five essential oils I bought were very basic: lavender, peppermint, geranium, orange and lemon. I started experimenting and blending and understanding the different known effects of each one, before graduating up to oils like sandalwood, juniper and pine and from that, the collection grew. But the idea in those early days was something relatively simple: it was finding a way to support my own wellbeing needs and to positively impact how I was feeling at that difficult time in my life.

I became really interested in the different known properties of the oils and how they would work together and I loved being able to create something a bit more bespoke and unique for myself and, after a while, for my friends, too. Primarily I started blending for my own anxiety, which was at an all-time high. Real Luxury is the first blend I created and is still one of our bestsellers today. It took me hundreds of attempts to get it just right – you can definitely smell the lavender, jasmine and sandalwood but there are actually up to twenty-four essential oils in there – and I see it as a cashmere blanket of a scent – cozy and comforting, but luxurious too. All these years on, it's still what I still reach for in the moments I need to create some calm. And that's how NEOM began – experimenting with different blends in mixing bowls in my kitchen and the tiny bathroom of my flat, the whole place smelling like an old apothecary. I had no idea that it would lead me here, writing this book. Of course, we've come a long way since then and over the years our blends have become more sophisticated and complex. We now work with different aromatherapists and perfumers, as well as having a product development team.

We're known for our scents, but I wouldn't call NEOM just a fragrance brand. It's not just about our blends smelling beautiful; our products have to work on multiple levels and help to deliver tangible wellbeing benefits too. We spent a long time devising what I think are the ultimate blends. Now the focus is to delve deeper into those categories to find new ways we can use our fragrances to help support people's sleep, stress, energy and mood needs. It's about how those oils can work in conjunction with any other wellbeing practices and exercises to help you.

'Our products have to work on multiple levels and help to deliver tangible wellbeing benefits.'

Where our products are concerned, it's about high quality, complex blends, tested products and the most appropriate inclusion of 100% natural essential oils, extracts and isolates. We put up to twenty-four essential oils in every blend and our signature 3-wick candles contain the equivalent of three to four 10ml essential oil bottles in every candle. Quite often we've worked with hundreds of different blends to find the exact one that's going to work in the best possible way and give the best results. We're also very keen on making sure that we communicate how that routine and regime is used, so people get the best possible benefits from it. We're passionate about creating products that respond to how people are *really* feeling and give them what they need to improve their wellbeing, which is why I'm so excited to share more about what I've learned over the years in this book.

As a brand that uses 100% natural fragrance and naturally derived ingredients, sustainability is at the heart of the business. Following a two-year process, we are a certified 'B Corporation' (or B Corp), which means we're part of a global community of businesses that meet high standards of social and environmental impact – it's about our people and planet, not just the bottom line! Becoming B Corp Certified is something I'm massively proud of, but for me it's really where we should all be moving towards as business leaders. That means everything from the suppliers, traceability and visibility on where everything comes from, through to the people who work for you and the culture that we're creating. That was baked into the business from the start; I think if you're interested in looking after yourself from a wellbeing point of view, it stands to reason you'd be interested in looking after people and the planet. Our 'north star' has always been to boost the wellbeing of our customers and community and now more than ever our planet needs us to.

It's not been without its challenges when it comes to essential oils. We've had to flex at times to change blends and redevelop fragrances if something is no longer sustainable. That's something that we do as a business and keep our eyes wide open to.

We have to evolve and change constantly. This is also why we've worked hard to ensure that this book is as sustainably produced as possible. In accordance with Penguin's commitment to the planet, this book has been created with the environment in mind. We have lessened its carbon impact by printing with a low-carbon FSC™ certified paper based in Sweden. All copies are printed locally in Suffolk, UK, using 100% renewable energy. Once you've read this book, we encourage you to re-gift it, or keep it for future reading! Alternatively, you can donate it to charity for someone else to enjoy or recycle it by checking with your local council or using www.recyclenow.com.

MY HERO ESSENTIAL OIL

If you invest in one essential oil, I think lavender is a good option. It's probably the most versatile oil – depending on the quantities and how it's used, it's known to be stimulating but also balancing. It works in lots of different ways, so it's a great go-to.

MY NEOM WORKHORSE

My most hardworking NEOM blend is Perfect Night's Sleep, no question. As I've said, to me sleep is the bedrock of all wellbeing and using Perfect Night's Sleep is a routine that I try and stick to every night. If I've got more time, I will be using multiple products from the Perfect Night's Sleep range like the Perfect Night's Sleep Candle, Bath Foam and Magnesium Body Butter, whereas my 'light' version of this when I'm travelling is just using the Perfect Night's Sleep Pillow Mist.

A Beginner's Guide to Essential Oils

I've talked a lot about my journey to discovering these oils and why I love them, but there is a lot more to these than meets the eye. So many of our customers want to know more about what they are, where they come from and how they work, so here is a bit of a deeper dive into these powerful substances, based on the most common questions I get asked.

What exactly are essential oils?

Essential oils are natural compounds extracted from parts of certain aromatic plants, flowers and trees. Each of these compounds has its own unique fragrance and active, volatile ingredients. Essential oils can be extracted from various parts, including the flowers, leaves, bark, resin, stem, fruit, seeds and roots. They're called essential oils because they contain the 'essence' of a plant and its unique fragrance.

What is the extraction process?

Extraction is mainly done through two methods: steam-based distillation, where steam is used to lift the delicate aroma from the plant (typically used for herbs and more botanical scents); and a mechanical 'cold' expression, where little or no heat is used (a process mainly used for citrus fruits, where the peel is punctured and the essential oil is pressed out).

On a biological level, how do essential oils boost our wellbeing?

Essential oils are made up of phytochemicals. Phytochemicals play a number of important roles in the body's immune and nervous systems, as well as reducing stress, fighting oxidative stress and cell damage, and being good for digestive, cardiovascular and respiratory health. Essential oils also interact directly with the neurotransmitters in our brain that are responsible for regulating our emotions.

How does that work?

Through a process called olfaction, which is basically our sense of smell. When you inhale essential oils, they are received by 50 million receptors in your olfactory system – the parts of your nose that enable you to smell. The olfactory system then sends signals to the limbic system in the brain. This is the part that manages emotional and behavioural responses, where it cleverly produces neurochemicals and hormones, which act like little messengers to help spark certain feelings.

Different essential oils bring different benefits, whether that's calming essential oils known to help relieve stress and feelings of tension that can be caused by anxiety; relaxing ones known to help you prepare for a perfect night's sleep; energizing ones known to boost energy; or uplifting ones known to help with your mood.

HOW ESSENTIAL OILS WORK

STIMULATE
THESE RECEPTORS THEN SEND A SIGNAL TO
YOUR LIMBIC SYSTEM – THE PART OF YOUR
BRAIN WHICH MANAGES EMOTIONAL AND
BEHAVIOURAL RESPONSES, WHERE IT CLEVERLY
PRODUCES NEUROCHEMICALS AND HORMONES

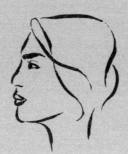

INHALE
WHEN YOU BREATHE IN
ESSENTIAL OILS, THEY ARE
RECEIVED BY 50 MILLION
RECEPTORS IN YOUR
OLFACTORY SYSTEM – THE
PART OF YOUR NOSE THAT
ENABLES YOU TO SMELL

RESPOND
THESE NEUROCHEMICALS
AND HORMONES THEN
ACT LIKE LITTLE MESSENGERS
TO HELP SPARK CERTAIN
FEELINGS

What essential oil is best for me? Is there one that's good for everyone?

Everyone has their own likes and dislikes and the same oil can have different effects on people. If you're drawn towards a particular scent, it's very likely that particular oil has the aromatherapeutic properties you need at that particular moment. NEOM's Scent Discovery Test is made up of four different scents, and whichever one is the most appealing to you can indicate your current wellbeing need.

Can essential oils work in other ways than inhalation?

There are some small studies that suggest essential oils can be absorbed through the barrier of the skin and into the bloodstream but this can depend on a whole mix of factors including things like temperature, exposure time and surface area. Essential oil is incredibly potent and applying it directly to the skin is not normally advised, to avoid potential irritation, so dilute in a carrier or base product if you're using them yourself. Because of their high potency, ingesting essential oils internally is not advised because of the potential side effects. Some essential oils are also phototoxic (including citrus oils), which means if you are applying essential oils to the skin you should not expose yourself to sunlight or other forms of ultraviolet light immediately afterwards, as it can cause a reaction or irritation.

Are essential oils the answer for everything?
As with anything related to health and wellbeing, essential oils certainly aren't the silver bullet or miracle solution for everything. But, used alongside a healthy lifestyle and following the appropriate medical advice if needed, they can be a natural and effective way to boost our everyday wellbeing.

What should I look out for in an essential oil?
For the highest grade, natural products look for what percentage is natural, amd what percentage is diluted in a carrier oil, as well as full details of the ingredients. Do a bit of digging into a brand to make sure their ingredients are sustainably sourced (their social media is a good place to start). Also, look at price points as they vary widely. Things like rose, sandalwood, frankincense and jasmine are

among the most expensive essential oils as they're more difficult to produce (for example, it takes approximately 10,000 rose blossoms to make one 5ml bottle of essential oil). If they're sitting at the cheaper end of the market they're probably not going to be natural or the best quality product, or they could be diluted heavily by a carrier oil.

MY GO-TO
WELLBEING TOOLKIT

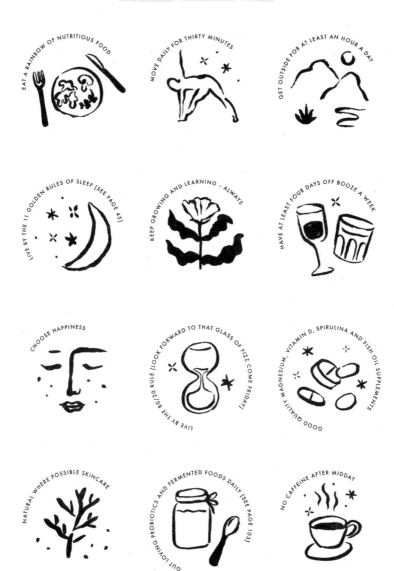

EAT A RAINBOW OF NUTRITIOUS FOOD

MOVE DAILY FOR THIRTY MINUTES

GET OUTSIDE FOR AT LEAST AN HOUR A DAY

LIVE BY THE 11 GOLDEN RULES OF SLEEP [SEE PAGE 45]

KEEP GROWING AND LEARNING – ALWAYS

HAVE AT LEAST FOUR DAYS OFF BOOZE A WEEK

CHOOSE HAPPINESS

LIVE BY THE 80/20 RULE [LOOK FORWARD TO THAT GLASS OF FIZZ COME FRIDAY]

GOOD QUALITY MAGNESIUM, VITAMIN D, SPIRULINA AND FISH OIL SUPPLEMENTS

NATURAL WHERE POSSIBLE SKINCARE

GUT LOVING PROBIOTICS AND FERMENTED FOODS DAILY [SEE PAGE 103]

NO CAFFEINE AFTER MIDDAY

MY AM TO PM
NEOM WELLBEING WONDERS

* **ENERGY**: Powered by 100% natural spearmint, rosemary and eucalyptus essential oils, the Super Shower Power Body Cleanser is the best way to set me up for the day.
* **MOOD**: Happiness Scented Candle – with a blend of up to ten essential oils including white neroli, mimosa and zingy lemon, I light this to give me a little lift.
* **STRESS**: Real Luxury Magnesium Body Butter – contains 88mg of magnesium in every 5ml and is super moisturizing. I love to slather this on post-bath.
* **SLEEP**: Perfect Night's Sleep Pillow Mist – my absolute bedtime go-to wherever I am. A few spritzes and I'm ready for bed.

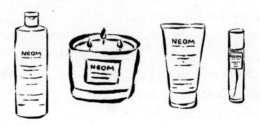

IT'S JUST MY OPINION, BUT . . .

WELLNESS FADS

Before we go any further, I thought it would be helpful to talk about what doesn't work as much as what does. It's something I get asked a lot and while I'm not a health expert, my two decades in the wellness industry have given me a pretty good steer on the supposed miracle answers and health shakes that promise to change your life overnight. I also appreciate that when we want to feel better we can feel driven to try lots of things, so as I mentioned previously with stress, if you're really struggling in any area I would advise you to visit your GP or a trusted health professional.

This 'No BS approach' has always informed the way I think about wellbeing and is what underpins the whole ethos of this book. What I mean by that is that, just like you, I have a busy life with all sorts of factors that can detract from my wellbeing, so I want to know that the things I choose to spend my time and money on are going to be worth it. I always look to quality, well-researched sources for advice and try to separate the facts from the fads, so that everything I put out there on socials, in our products and in this book are worth your time too. I would advise you to do the same as you embark on your own wellbeing journey and start to try different things in your own toolkit. Try to keep your own lifestyle in mind and only take on board the advice that really applies to you. Ultimately, I think it's about using a bit of common sense and – when in doubt – trusting expert advice and science-backed products that make you feel better and not worse (or no different!). Here are some of the latest trends that, personally, I'm not a fan of.

1. **Charcoal detoxing**. It's become super popular in food and supplements but I personally don't really believe in products that promise to 'detoxify'. This is the primary function of our liver so the body should be able to detoxify itself naturally anyway.

2. **Blue-light-blocking glasses**. The idea is that they block out the blue light that technology and some lights emit, which in turn helps us get better sleep and make our circadian rhythm work better (read more about circadian rhythms on page 44). Why not just turn down the lights and steer clear of technology in the evenings? I think we're fighting an unnecessary battle there.

3. **Juice cleanses**. I think they can be helpful sometimes if you need to kick start a healthy eating spurt, but they're just not sustainable. It's quite hardcore, they can be very expensive and, essentially, it's a crash diet that's packaged up as something healthy. I think you should just nourish the body with really good whole foods for a week, rather than not eating solid foods at all.

4. **Over supplementing**. Given how much the supplement industry is booming at the moment, the tendency

can be there to take a whole load of supplements in the hope it will fix all our problems (better skin, energy, gut health). But, we should really be getting the majority of our nutrients from the food that we eat, and supplements can't replace a good, varied diet. I'm not against them if they're really great quality and are right for you (see more on this on page 195); I'm just against people using them as a supplement – excuse the pun – for eating and drinking the right things.

5. **Sauna blankets**. This is an odd one for me. If you want to recreate that experience, just go and sit in a sauna – most local leisure centres or gyms have them, which you can often visit with just a day pass. I can't understand why anyone would spend a fortune on a blanket that gets you all sweaty and which you've got to get out and pump up in your own home, and then clean again before putting away. That seems like a crazy and inconvenient expense to me.

6. **Energy workout drinks**. We're told that they will help us fuel our bodies but so many of them are formulated with sugars and stimulants that aren't good for us. Most of them are really poor quality and, in fact, we just need to drink more water – so just save the money, ditch the stimulants and fill up your bottle!

7. **Natural sugars**. They've become really widely available and are marketed as a healthy alternative to refined sugar. However, the term 'natural sugar' is hugely misleading and there's no real difference in the body's processing of natural sweeteners compared to refined

sugars. All sweeteners, whether it's agave syrup or white sugar, are pretty much equal. Sugar is sugar!

8. **Hardcore workouts**. Obviously, moving our body is important for wellbeing but I'm not a fan of exercising too much or too intensely. High intensity workouts can have their place, but the research shows that extreme exercise can affect our hormones negatively and put extra stress on our adrenal glands, which especially isn't great if we're exercising to try and bring down our stress levels! Moderate exercise done consistently and trying to generally be as active as possible is what works for me.

9. **Restrictive diets**. For example, the keto diet, which is high fat, low carb. These diets do have their place if you've got a medical condition, but essentially the way people use the diet is often in a fasting scenario, which you can't maintain for very long. Getting enough good carbs from fruit and veg is one of the main components of healthy eating.

TIPS ON HOW TO USE THIS BOOK

THINK HOLISTICALLY

You might intrinsically feel that you have just one of the 'four pillar' issues that you want to address first, and that's fine. But it's also worth keeping an open mind, as your underlying wellbeing needs might be different to what you think they are. A case in point is our Scent Discovery Test, which we encourage customers to do at the start of their NEOM journey. This involves inhaling four different vials based around each of our pillars to discover which one they're drawn to the most. A high percentage of people who do the test find their wellbeing needs are caused by something else. For example, someone might come in feeling tired and wanting an energy boost, but because they're not exercising or going outside during day light hours this in turn affects their sleep, which makes them feel even more tired, which affects their mood and so on. So it's more about addressing the root cause rather than the presenting symptom, and knowing that one thing is generally linked to another. Feel free to go straight to the chapter on the pillar you feel you need the most help with, but also bear in mind that for the vast majority of people it's often coming from somewhere different.

NEOM BLENDS

As we've already mentioned, NEOM uses 100% natural essential oils and the blends are central to everything we do. It's important to understand their benefits and how they can complement the rest of the advice in the book, so when I recommend certain products, they'll make sense to a particular wellbeing need.

THE PRACTICALS

Before you start, you might want to think about what – or who – else might help you on your wellbeing journey. I recommend using a journal to record your thoughts or track your progress. It could be something else like upgrading your pillows for something plumper, or investing in a new water bottle that you will remember to take with you and enjoy drinking from. But I would say that the most important thing in your toolkit is your mindset. Have a kind, can-do attitude towards yourself and you'll be off to the best start possible and will set the tone to really enjoy the ride along the way.

TWEAK AS NEEDED

In the same way that we might plan ahead for things like work and holidays, I think we should make our wellbeing journey something we're constantly aware of. How are we doing with that wellbeing toolkit? Does anything need tweaking or changing? It's not about chastising yourself but just being aware and focusing your energy on what you might need to turn up a bit, or tone down. As I often say, it's not about completely overhauling your life and chucking the baby out with the bathwater, but rather making small tweaks in the here and now.

THE 80/20 RULE

I'm a big believer in the 80/20 rule, which is about living a realistic life rather than one of deprivation. Look after yourself and implement the changes that you need (80 per cent of the time), but don't be afraid to enjoy a glass of fizz (or two) come Friday (the remaining 20 per cent). You'll find no preaching here!

WELLBEING EXPERTS

I've been lucky to work with some of the best experts over the years, who are all thought leaders in their own fields. Many of them are featured in this book and they've shared their wisdom and the latest knowledge of cutting-edge science in ways that we can directly apply to our own lives, along with some great questions asked by our wellbeing community. For more information and further reading, you'll find all the experts listed in my Little Black Book of Wellbeing (see page 241), along with the references cited in this book (see page 257).

1.
SLEEP

I was a great sleeper for most of my life. I was the kind of kid who could sleep in a car, in a plane, I never needed a particular mattress, I slept well in central London, in the countryside . . . nothing was a problem. It was only when I hit forty a few years ago that I started to struggle with my sleep. This could be down to a number of factors: hormones, more stress and responsibility, or simply that the bedroom's too hot, but modern life is also unfortunately perpetuating bad sleep for quite a few reasons.

Adults in developed countries like the UK and US spend up to 90 per cent of their day, around 22 hours, inside. This compares to 150 years ago, when people used to spend 90 per cent of their time *outside*. A survey of nearly 17,000 people in fifteen countries across Europe and North America found that people vastly underestimated how much time they spent inside, with one in six respondents saying they rarely went outdoors. We are now what's been called the 'Indoor Generation', a technologically advanced society with convenience and mod cons at our disposal, but at the sacrifice of natural daylight and fresh air. For lots of people these days their commute consists of a short walk to the living room. We work, shop, socialize and work out online and while there are obvious advantages, we just don't get outside as much as we used to and it's potentially contributing to a whole host of problems.

And none more than when it comes to sleep and the disruption of our circadian rhythms. These internal timers are set to a 24-hour cycle and are present in all of life. In humans our circadian rhythm plays a vital role in keeping our physical, mental and behavioural systems in a state of equilibrium, known as homeostasis. Circadian rhythms affect everything from our sleep and immune systems to hormones, metabolism, appetite and mood. Crucially, they are reset by following the natural light/dark cycle. Thanks to research in this field, we're fast realizing that getting enough daylight is essential for our health and wellbeing. We'll be looking into it further and discovering the 'best' type of daylight later on in the chapter.

If we can nail our sleep it can have such a positive impact on all other areas of our lives. We have more energy to do our jobs and look after our families, our moods aren't impacted as much by stressful events, we become more resilient and we're just more available to enjoy life. There's no point having a cupboard full of supplements or an expensive gym membership that you never use if you're tired, overwhelmed and exhausted all the time.

I'm really not an evangelist in any other areas, but sleep is the one thing I take quite seriously. I think this is partly because, unfortunately for me, I'm not the sort of person who can mess around with their sleep too much without suffering the consequences, so I always make sure I'm in bed by 10pm. I read a book for half an hour to decompress and the lights are off by half past ten. I'm quite religious about that. If I'm really into watching something I will occasionally stay up later but with the knowledge that I won't feel my best the next day. For me, that is usually an incentive to switch off and go to bed.

So, it's about having those little moments of discipline

sometimes, but also not overcomplicating matters. If there's going to be any mantras in this book, it's this one. Sleep is the gateway to better wellbeing!

As I've got older, the effects of not getting enough sleep aren't something I can brush off any more. The outcome is much more dramatic on my lifestyle. I'll really notice that I'm not in a good mood, or I'm feeling stressed out about things that wouldn't bother me otherwise; if I feel unwell from lack of sleep I'll be cancelling plans . . . the list goes on. On the upside, I do need a bit less sleep now I'm older (read about how our age affects how much sleep we need on page 54). It just has to be *quality* sleep. I think the main takeaway here is about having an ongoing awareness of how we are sleeping and making adjustments when we need to.

THE 11 GOLDEN RULES
FOR BETTER SLEEP

It turns out I'm not the only one whose sleep has taken a turn for the worse. My friends are talking about poor sleep more than ever and the general consensus is that everyone seems to be sleeping worse, whether it's down to our age, work, stress, health, family responsibilities or just managing the juggle of life. There's so much more noise about sleep now and consequently, a lot more information out there. Which is good because we're acknowledging the importance of it, but on the other hand it can all feel a bit confusing and overwhelming. That was how the idea for the 11 Golden Rules was born. It doesn't matter what age you are or what's going on in your life, I know from my own sleep journey, and hearing about other people's, how much we'd benefit from a science-backed, easy-to-follow and super powerful 'all you need to know' guide to better sleep. So that's what we created.

The 11 Golden Rules for Better Sleep were devised by the NEOM team and top sleep specialist and performance coach Nick Witton. I describe Nick as the conduit between academia and the real world. He's at the forefront of some super exciting stuff happening in the field of circadian neuroscience and in particular the role daylight plays in our sleep. It's a massively emerging field and one that we'll be hearing lots more about in the years to come. Nick has helped us to distil a decade's worth of experience and cutting-edge research into a very NEOM, user-friendly 'small steps' approach.

And trust me, the Golden Rules really do work. Since I started following them, I have been sleeping brilliantly and I've now got this amazing maintenance plan for life. I've been blown away by the amount of people who've got in touch to say how much better their sleep is; for many, they're sleeping the best they ever have. Ninety-four per cent saw their sleep improve after just one week following this plan.*

HOW TO DO THEM

The Rules are designed to be followed over a 28-day period, which I find is the time it usually takes to turn a new habit into an automatic behaviour. It is a commitment, so to get the most out of the plan it's best that you follow the rules every day. But sometimes things don't go to plan, so remember that we're aiming for progress, not perfection. They might take a bit of get-ting used to but stick with it. Personally, I found not drinking alcohol 3 hours before bed a bit hard at first, as well as getting out into daylight first thing, but I really have noticed a massive

* External independent blind study on 107 volunteers for two weeks.

difference in my sleep and energy levels from doing it. If you do fall off the wagon with any of them, just get back on it the next day.

'The secret to success with this is consistency and practising all 11 Rules together. Keep at it for the 28 days as this is the prime time for you to form new habits.'

– Nick Witton

SLEEP is the gateway to better wellbeing

THE 11 GOLDEN RULES
FOR BETTER SLEEP

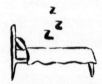

1. GO TO BED **THE SAME TIME** EVERY NIGHT AND GET UP AT THE **SAME TIME** EVERY MORNING – EVEN AT WEEKENDS.

2. SLEEP IN **90-MINUTE CYCLES** SO YOU EITHER AIM FOR 7½, 9 OR 10½ HOURS SLEEP.

3. **DON'T SNOOZE** YOUR ALARM.

4. GIVE YOURSELF **30 MINUTES TO WAKE UP** EACH MORNING.

'The secret to success with this is consistency and practising all 11 Rules together. Keep at it for the 28 days as this is the prime time for you to form new habits.'

NICK WITTON

5. GET AT LEAST **1 HOUR OF DIRECT SUNLIGHT** (OUTSIDE OR SITTING BY A WINDOW) BEFORE MIDDAY, IDEALLY 15 MINUTES OF THESE WITHIN THE FIRST HOUR OF WAKING.

6. DO AT LEAST **30 MINUTES OF MOVEMENT** A DAY.

7. CREATE AN EVENING ROUTINE: USE THE **3,2,1 RULE EVERY NIGHT**. 3 HOURS BEFORE BED – NO FOOD OR ALCOHOL. 2 HOURS BEFORE BED – NO WORK OR STRENUOUS EXERCISE. 1 HOUR BEFORE BED – NO SCREENS AND DIM THE LIGHTS.

8. SET ASIDE **15 MINUTES FOR RELAXATION** AT ANY POINT IN YOUR DAY (WHATEVER THAT MEANS TO YOU).

9. MAKE YOUR BEDROOM **A TECH-FREE ZONE** THAT'S AS DARK AS POSSIBLE AND BETWEEN 16 and 19°C.

10. EAT **THREE REGULAR MEALS** EVENLY SPREAD OUT THROUGHOUT THE DAY.

11. HAVE **YOUR LAST COFFEE** (OR CAFFEINATED DRINK) BY **MIDDAY**.

RULE 1:
Go to bed at the same time every night and get up at the same time every morning – even at weekends

WHY?

Our bodies love routine. This especially applies to our sleep patterns and sticking to a regular wake-up time and bedtime helps to strengthen the timing of our circadian rhythm. Well-regulated circadian rhythms are essential for achieving good-quality sleep, as well as the length of time it takes us to fall asleep, which is called sleep latency.

Our wake and sleep times can vary throughout our lives but there's a pretty standard way most of us 'do' sleep. The average person is put into a routine by a caregiver pretty soon after they're born. Through childhood we have set bedtimes and school to get up for, along with weekend schedules for things like sports and activities. Our sleep schedules might start to waver if we go to university or do shift work, as do 15 per cent of the UK population, but in adult life our jobs become our main marker for when we get up and go to bed, especially in the week.

My wake-up time has been pretty consistent for the past fifteen years. A full-time job and raising children means that I pretty much wake up (and get up) around 7am. Evenings are a different ball game. It's harder to ring-fence your bedtime when you don't have anywhere specific to be the next morning (i.e. at your desk, doing the school drop-off). Think about what your own evenings might currently look like. You might be out late seeing friends, catching up on emails, flicking through social media, or binge-watching something to switch off. If we tried to tip our kids or own childhood selves into bed after all that and said,

'Off you go to sleep then,' chances are it's not going to happen and it's exactly the same with our adult selves!

It's not always achievable to get up and go to bed at exactly the same time every day, but evidence shows that people who stick to a regular sleep–wake cycle report feeling more alert for longer periods in the day and sleep for longer (and better) at night. Even losing one hour of sleep over a few days can have an effect, say studies, and lead to a decrease in performance, mood and thinking. Unsurprisingly, children who have regular bed-times are found to perform better in tests for memory, attention, inhibition and cognitive functions like multitasking. No matter how old we are, we could all probably benefit from some sort of bedtime routine.

SMASHING A SLEEP MYTH:
'I'LL JUST CATCH UP ON SLEEP AT THE WEEKEND'

It's a common belief that if we miss out on sleep in the week, we can just catch up on the deficit at the weekends with a lie-in. Unfortunately, the reality isn't that simple. Rather than topping up as and when, we have specific times for different phases of sleep and each of those phases performs a different function. 'Sleep isn't like money, where you'd save different amounts on different days and end up with the same total at the end of the week,' says sleep expert Nick Witton.

If we sleep for say, 5 hours on a weeknight and 12 hours at the weekend, we may still have the same total amount of sleep at the end of the week as if we'd slept evenly for 18 hours, but the quality of our sleep will be different. Restricted sleep will cause a dearth in the amount of REM sleep, which is vital for recovery and memory retention, while with too much sleep the beneficial effects rapidly diminish as each hour goes by. Varied sleep times can lead to something called social jet lag. It has been reported that a third of us experience 2 hours or more of social jet lag, which is equivalent to flying from London to New York each week and flying back for the weekend. 'Social jet lag is a real thing,' says Nick. 'We need to be more aware of it.'

First coined in 2006, 'social jet lag' is the specific term to describe people who under sleep in the week and over sleep at weekends. This causes our melatonin (the sleep-inducing hormone) and cortisol (the alerting hormone) to become out of sync, which upsets the cycle of our natural body clock. Research shows that people who sleep for longer periods at the weekend often feel more tired during weekdays. Those suffering from social jet lag are also more likely to experience bad moods, while a Brazilian study on 4,051 adults (67 per cent of whom were female) found that respondents who experienced 2 hours or more of social jet lag were more likely to experience depressive symptoms.

WHY LACK OF SLEEP MAKES US 'METABOLICALLY GROGGY'

An irregular sleep schedule can affect our metabolism and result in burning fewer calories at rest (also known as RMR or Resting Metabolic Rate). Sleep deprivation interferes with our insulin levels, the hormone needed to change sugar, starch and other food into energy for our body. This makes us 'metabolically groggy', says a study from Chicago University, as our bodies have trouble processing this blood sugar (also known as glucose) into our bloodstream and cells, instead storing them as fat. And when we have less energy, evidence also shows we're also more likely to reach for the higher-calorie, carb-dense foods (read more about how sleep affects our hunger hormones on page 226), so you can see how unhelpful cycles can start.

Set yourself a regular bedtime and wake-up time and keep to it, even at weekends (within 30 minutes). Rising at the same time, or as close to it as possible, is one of the most powerful anchors to keep our circadian rhythm functioning regularly (and keep social jet lag at bay). Don't stress if it doesn't always work out, the odd late night is part of life, but just be mindful that it doesn't become a regular thing.

EAT AND EXERCISE AT THE SAME TIME

This is particularly important if your schedule doesn't allow you to get enough sleep. Keeping these specific routines consistent offers a cue for your circadian rhythms to stay on track. It's better to exercise early in the day, as exercise increases both our cortisol levels and core temperature, neither of which make great bedfellows. You can read more about the benefits of exercise on our sleep in Rule 6.

SLEEP CHRONOTYPES

A sleep chronotype is the term used to describe a person's personal body clock and will set an innate preference for timings of sleep and activity, or in basic terms what most of us understand as 'early birds' and 'night owls'. Unsurprisingly, early birds perform better both mentally and physically earlier on in the day, whereas night owls function at their best from late afternoon into the evening. Our chronotypes also vary with age. Children generally tend to be early types (no surprise there) but starting towards puberty, chronotype shifts more to an evening type, peaking at adolescence – hence those morning battles getting teenagers out of bed. As we enter adulthood our chronotype generally goes back to an earlier morning type. Traditionally night owls have always been more likely to be out of sync with the 9–5 working hours during the week, but the rise of flexible working means we have more chance to work in line with our natural body clocks (but also work later, which isn't always a good thing!). So, if you struggle to get up in the mornings or feel tired whatever time you go to bed, it could be that you're sleeping against your chronotype.

TRIAL SLEEP TIMES

If the above sounds like you, I would suggest trying different sleep and wake times (regardless of what others do) until you find out what works for you. Try and prioritize your sleep as much as you can. If you've always struggled in the mornings regardless of circumstance and would benefit from an extra hour in bed in the morning, why not ask if you can come into work a bit later and finish later instead? We thankfully live in an era of flexi working, so it makes sense to make the most of our sleep chronotype. It's not about being 'lazy' but finding a schedule that best suits you, so you will be at your best and most productive. Unsure what your best wake and sleep times are? Rule 2 will help with that.

RULE 2:
Sleep in 90-minute cycles, aiming for 7½, 9 or 10½ hours

WHY?

Probably *the* biggest misconception is that we should all be sleeping for eight uninterrupted hours a night. The reality is that the 8 hours we've been taught to aim for is simply because the government guidelines suggest 7 to 9 hours and eight is slap-bang in the middle. However, just like most things in life, and certainly when it comes to wellbeing, there is no 'one size fits all' model for sleep.

> **'Like most things in life,
> and certainly when it comes to wellbeing,
> there is no "one size fits all" model for sleep.'**

Rather than sleeping in one long stretch, we actually sleep in cycles. Nighttime sleep is made up of several rounds of these cycles, each of which is composed of four different stages. In a typical night a person goes through four to six sleep cycles, each of which lasts for approximately 90 minutes. Sleep cycles can differ night to night and vary on things like a person's age, hormones and the time of the month, stress, alcohol consumption and when we last had caffeine.

We also have different types of sleep. Sleep is made up of two neurological states: NREM (non rapid eye movement) and REM (rapid eye movement). We alternate between these light and deep states throughout the night. Deep sleep occurs primarily in the first half of the night. As the night goes on, these stages get shorter

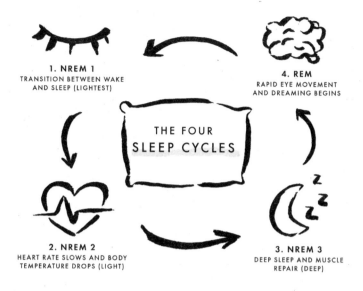

1. NREM 1
TRANSITION BETWEEN WAKE
AND SLEEP (LIGHTEST)

4. REM
RAPID EYE MOVEMENT
AND DREAMING BEGINS

THE FOUR
SLEEP CYCLES

2. NREM 2
HEART RATE SLOWS AND BODY
TEMPERATURE DROPS (LIGHT)

3. NREM 3
DEEP SLEEP AND MUSCLE
REPAIR (DEEP)

and we spend more time in REM sleep, before going into a light sleep stage prior to waking up.

WHY IS DEEP SLEEP IMPORTANT?

Deep sleep is when brain activity slows down and our bodily processes kick in. This stage is essential for recovery and growth, as well as bolstering the immune system and other key processes like collagen production. It's also good for our minds: a 2022 Cambridge University study found a link between cognitive decline and disrupted deeper slow wave sleep. This is because deep sleep is neuroprotective (also known as a 'deep clean' for the brain) and helps the brain get rid of certain toxins, including the build-up of a protein called amyloid. Studies show that deep sleep is important for both our short- and long-term memory, and how we process the information we learned that day. This helps free up space in our brain to take in new stuff, which in turn sharpens our focus and increases our learning.

REM

The REM, or rapid eye movement, stage is when our brains get busy again. This is the stage where the most vivid dreams happen, caused by the rapid uptake in brain activity. REM is widely believed to be essential for cognitive functions like learning, memory and creativity, or in particular, what experts call 'creative problem solving'. This is because it's thought REM time allows the brain time to roam freely and form connections between previously unrelated ideas.

Have you ever woken up from a really weird or bonkers dream after a night out? Drinking alcohol decreases REM sleep early in the night but as the effects wear off there's an REM rebound, which pushes the REM stages later into the sleep cycle. So that last sambuca shot really can be the stuff of nightmares!

RULE 3:
Don't snooze your alarm

WHY?

How do you wake up in the mornings? Are you a 'spring out of bed as soon as your alarm goes off' type person, or is it more of a case of hitting the snooze button and going back to sleep?

Many of us have an on–off relationship with the snooze button – quite literally. A recent study by the University of Notre Dame looked at the sleep habits of adults in full-time employment. It found that six out of ten respondents hit the snooze button in the mornings, while 57 per cent habitually slept in. When respondents were able to wake up naturally, they usually slept longer and consumed less caffeine in the day.

Hitting snooze is standard behaviour in the mornings, with a commonly held view that it's the best way to wake up. But studies say the opposite and rather than easing us into the day, it can actually have a knock-on effect. Fight or flight mode is our automatic physiological response to a stressful event and our bodies release the stress hormone cortisol to deal with the perceived threat. That can include being woken up suddenly by a loud noise such as our alarm; every time we hit that snooze button, we're in danger of cranking up the stress levels even further. And snoozing doesn't even really work: the average pause between snoozes is between 5 and 10 minutes, which is not enough time for us to drop back into a restorative sleep.

WHAT'S THE ALTERNATIVE?

In an ideal world we'd be waking up naturally. With our melatonin levels low, our cortisol production naturally surges just before we wake, which is why we feel alert and refreshed after a good night's sleep. We can work out our natural wake-up time according to how many sleep cycles we need (see Rule 2).

However, modern life dictates that most of us need outside help to wake up at a certain time, especially for the night owl chronotypes who have a natural tendency to sleep later. Continue to set your alarm but resist the temptation to hit the snooze button; instead just get up. No matter how tired you might feel at first, tell yourself it's only temporary and that you know you will feel better once you're up and moving about. It's about forming a new habit and training yourself to get up, so your brain and body become used to it.

Also, think about what kind of alarm you use. Many of us use the standard alarm on our phones but try looking at more restful tones, like chimes or soft music. Or you might use a digital alarm clock that's tuned into your station of choice, whether it's the breakfast news, music, or relentlessly upbeat presenters in mid conversation. But rather than being the motivational kick-start we were perhaps hoping for, it can feel more like coming to in the middle of a noisy room. Look at more gentle 'rise and shines' that offer a less jarring wake-up. Lots of digital alarm clocks offer calming nature-based sounds, while wake-up lights that gradually lighten until they're fully lit are known to minimize sleep inertia, that groggy feeling we get when we're suddenly woken up out of a deep sleep (more on this in the next rule).

Ask me anything

Q: What do you think about sleep apps and trackers and would you recommend them?
A: I'm going to be controversial and say I am really not a fan of sleep tech. I don't need something telling me I've not had a great night's sleep – because I will usually know that already and it will only make me feel worse. There are also reports that it can make people feel worse to read that they had less than 7 hours of quality sleep the night before, even if they feel as though they slept well. Quality sleep is more important than the length of our sleep so I think that it can be problematic to track it. Not only that, becoming too fixated on any aspect of our health can lead to issues around control, which can ironically be detrimental to our overall wellbeing. I think the Calm app can be quite good for

some of the sleepy stories and meditations, so that's the only thing I would recommend.

RULE 4:
Give yourself 30 minutes to 'wake up' each morning

WHY?

Even if we're well rested and have timed our sleep cycles to perfection, it's rare for most of us to open our eyes and immediately spring out of bed first thing. This is because of something called 'sleep inertia', which is the transition period between sleep and wakefulness and is commonly known as the grogginess we feel upon awakening.

Sleep inertia is a normal biological process that generally lasts for anything from 15 minutes to an hour, but it can be longer, especially if you're a night owl chronotype, a shift worker or work other irregular hours. Sleep inertia is characterized by reduced reaction times, impaired visual attention and reduced cognitive abilities such as mathematical calculations – so it's probably not a good idea to go on your banking app and do any big transactions while still in bed!

Chronotype and sleep deprivation can both play a hand in sleep inertia but the big takeaway message here is to give yourself enough time to ease into the day. That doesn't mean lying in bed for longer though, as our minds start to form an association with being awake in bed, which can lead to unhelpful patterns when we do want to be asleep at night. So no matter how strong the urge to stay put under that nice warm duvet, it's best to get up and start moving gently, or stimulating our senses in other ways.

HOW?

Morning movement is a great way to wake up and set the tone for the day. Exercise increases the levels of the stimulating hormones cortisol and adrenaline, as well as suppressing the sleep-friendly hormone melatonin. It doesn't mean hitting a 5am HITT class (unless that is your thing); according to studies from Harvard University, even stretching can help wake up the body and improve circulation, which gets us set up for the day.

THINK PINK

Ever used the sound of an electrical appliance as a sleep aid? The repetitive humdrum of white noise is often touted as a good way to get off to sleep, but pink noise could be equally good for waking us up. Pink noise is more commonly nature-based sounds like waves crashing on a beach, rain falling and leaves rustling in trees. Small-scale studies have found that listening to pink noise first thing in the morning can reduce sleep inertia and improve spatial memory, which is what we need for remembering where we put things or recalling a route to a certain place. So instead of tuning into your normal radio station, trying a bit of pink noise in the morning could be a restful but rousing alternative instead.

MORNING JOURNALLING

As well as being good for creativity, journalling can be very cathartic and help us organize our thoughts, and has been linked to managing anxiety, reducing stress and even boosting physical health. Morning journalling can be a really good way to frame a positive mindset or set an intention for that day. If you're not sure how to go about it, check out the 'morning pages' exercise outlined in Julia Cameron's classic book, *The Artist's Way*. The process is super simple: just do three pages of a longhand stream of consciousness every morning. There's no right or wrong way to do it and the only rule is that it's for your eyes only!

RULE 5:
Get at least 1 hour of direct sunlight (outside or sitting by a window) before midday, ideally 15 minutes of these within the first hour of waking

WHY?

We've already touched on circadian rhythms, but light is one of the biggest factors in how they function within our bodies. To recap, they are the 24-hour cycles that run our internal body clock, carrying out essential functions and processes. One of the most important and well-known circadian rhythms is the sleep–wake cycle. The sleep–wake cycle follows a master 'clock' in the brain, which is directly influenced by outside environmental cues, the biggest of which is light. This basically means we know when to go outside and be awake and we know when it's dark and we should be asleep. The different hormones in our body that tell us to do these things will change accordingly throughout the 24-hour cycle, taking their cues from dawn and dusk.

THE CIRCADIAN CYCLE

Early doors
Our circadian clock is set every day by the rising of the sun, when the early morning blue rays of sunlight are at their most powerful

and alert our brains that the new day is here. Despite the bad press, blue light during the daytime is vital in syncing our body clocks to the outside world.

Daytime
Regular light exposure throughout the day causes the master clock to keep sending signals to our brain to keep us awake.

Evening time
As night falls and the sun goes down, our body's master clock initiates the production of melatonin. Melatonin levels start rising around 2 hours before our natural bedtime and, crucially, optimum production can only happen in dim light.

Circadian rhythms aren't just crucial for sleep. They also play a vital role in most vital bodily functions including metabolism, immune systems and heart health, and disrupted circadian rhythms have been linked to people with non-seasonal depression. Those who do have winter depression, which is the most common form of seasonal affective disorder (SAD), experience (unsurprisingly) severe depressive symptoms in the winter, followed by a remission in spring.

So circadian rhythms are a big deal. But as we discussed at the start of the chapter, modern life can disrupt them in a number of ways and a huge one is the lack of daylight. 'From all the research I've done over the years, the disconnect we see between the day and the night cycle to the outside world underpins a great number of physical and mental health problems, as well as a number of behaviours such as engagement, satisfaction, empathy and mood,' says Nick Witton. 'We've lost our fundamental connection to the outside world.'

'We've lost our fundamental connection to the outside world.'

– sleep expert Nick Witton

I think this is a bit of a game-changer, because it shifts our focus away from thinking that sleep is something that we can only influence at night, and can encourage us to have much more of a 360 approach. The simple act of stepping outside more often can have material pay-offs for all our wellbeing needs, but none so more than when it comes to sleep. Best of all, it's completely free!

> **Top tip:** If you need an extra boost in the mornings, take your morning wake up outdoors to get some exposure to that all important morning daylight. Try a stretch in the sun, shaking out your yoga mat on the patio or lawn for a quick routine, or going for a brisk walk around the block.

LET'S TALK ABOUT LIGHT

Although natural daylight might appear to be made of one clear colour, it is actually made up of the seven colours of the rainbow, along with invisible ultraviolet and ultrared light. All have different wavelengths: blue and violet have shorter wavelengths and are more intense, while colours like red and orange travel in longer waves and have less energy. We're often told about the negative effects of blue light exposure but not all blue light is bad. We get natural doses of blue light from the sun throughout the morning hours, which signals our body to wake up. While natural blue light is balanced out proportionally in the full spectrum of colours, artificial blue light is more concentrated and contains short, alerting rays which can overstimulate us if we have too much at the wrong time. The levels of blue light decrease as the day goes on until sunset, which is made up of mostly red, lower-level light. This red light triggers our body to increase melatonin levels and prepare for sleep. We'll hear more on the impact of artificial blue light in Rule 7, but the main takeaway here is simple – top up on more natural blue light first thing and avoid too much artificial blue light at night!

Ask me anything

Q: What do you think of SAD lamps? Do they work?
A: I think SAD lamps can be quite effective in the darker months when you're working for long stretches of time at your desk, but they should never take the place of natural daylight. If you're not sure which brand is best, it's worth doing your research: some brands use terms like 'medically certified' or 'medically approved', which means they've been recommended for use for a particular condition and have supported evidence.

LUX LEVELS

Light is measured in something called lux, which is a standardized unit for measuring illuminance and intensity. Lux levels vary massively between natural and artificial light, and also depending on what time of day and what month it is. A typical office has 300 lux, whereas even outside on the cloudiest day the reading will be around 10,000 lux. A bright sunny day in the middle of summer with a big blue sky is around 100,000 lux. Studies say

AVERAGE LUX LEVELS

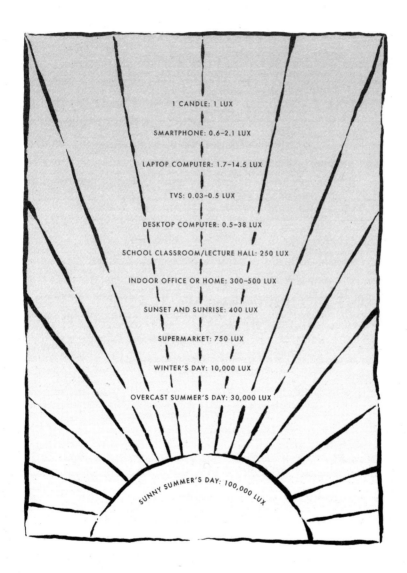

1 CANDLE: 1 LUX

SMARTPHONE: 0.6–2.1 LUX

LAPTOP COMPUTER: 1.7–14.5 LUX

TVS: 0.03–0.5 LUX

DESKTOP COMPUTER: 0.5–38 LUX

SCHOOL CLASSROOM/LECTURE HALL: 250 LUX

INDOOR OFFICE OR HOME: 300–500 LUX

SUNSET AND SUNRISE: 400 LUX

SUPERMARKET: 750 LUX

WINTER'S DAY: 10,000 LUX

OVERCAST SUMMER'S DAY: 30,000 LUX

SUNNY SUMMER'S DAY: 100,000 LUX

this is the ideal amount we need to sleep well. Conversely, most standard office lighting is around 500 lux or below.

A BIT ABOUT UV LIGHT

The sun emits three types of UV or ultraviolet radiation: UVA (ultraviolet A), UVB (ultraviolet B) and UVC (ultraviolet C), although UVC is blocked by the ozone layer and doesn't reach the earth's surface. UVA rays, on the other hand, penetrate further into the skin and contribute to long-term ageing, making up around 95 per cent of the UV rays that reach our skin. UVB rays are shorter and more intense, typically damaging the outer layers of the skin and causing sunburn. UVA rays are present all year round, even when it's winter or cloudy, while UVB radiation is strongest in the northern hemisphere between April and October. Although a double-glazed window will block most of the dangerous UVB rays, some UVA rays do get through. This is great for our body clock but natural light can be harmful to our skin in large quantities, so if you spend long periods of time by a window or in the conservatory, take precautions, such as wearing a full-spectrum sunscreen or a hat with a peak or wide brim.

HOW TO DO IT

Out of all the rules, getting outside first thing was one of the hardest for me. I've got kids, a dog, a busy job and messages that always need to be answered – half the morning can run away before I've even looked up outside at the sky. So I thought it would be hard, but actually making a concerted effort has really made a big difference to a) my energy levels during the day and b) how well I sleep that night. It's just something I now do without even thinking about it and the pay-off has been quite incredible.

A 30-minute walk every morning is the perfect way to start my day but it's not always logistically possible. If I can't do that, I'll make little tweaks. I always like a cup of tea in bed first thing but now I get up and have it in the kitchen, which is the sunniest spot in the house. In the summer, I'll go outside for my meetings or to make a phone call instead of staying at my desk. Any activity that I can feasibly move outside or by a natural light source, I will. So even if you're having one of those days where you haven't been able to leave the house or office, something as simple as sitting by a window to have your cup of tea or coffee is still a wellbeing win and will increase the amount of daylight you get without any major effort on your part.

Other ways to get light into your day:

* Eat breakfast or have your morning coffee outside.
* Do your morning make-up/beauty routine by a window.
* Sit by a window (or two ideally) to make phone calls or to do life admin.
* Work from home? Move your desk/workstation to where you get more natural light.
* Get out at lunchtime – even if it's just a quick walk around the block.
* Create a peaceful 'sun spot' in your house where you can sit and read, or do a mindfulness activity like meditation.
* Short on time in the mornings? Get off the bus one stop early on your commute or park the car further away from the office.

* Go for a 'walk and talk' meeting to get that extra 30 minutes of daylight.
* Swap the gym for exercising in the garden/park once a week.

RULE 6:
Do at least 30 minutes of exercise (or some form of movement) daily

WHY?

Studies have shown that how we move in the day (and how much) is critical to how well we sleep at night. Aside from the obvious health benefits, a daily movement practice helps us to a) fall asleep quicker and b) sleep for longer. *When* we do it is also key. As I mentioned earlier, getting moving first thing boosts our levels of serotonin, cortisol and feel-good endorphins (aka our happy hormones), as well as regulating our circadian rhythms and sleep–wake–sleep cycle. For the same reasons, we should avoid doing anything too strenuous or any exercise with loud music pumping later on or at night.

New guidelines set in 2020 by the World Health Organization recommended that all adults should undertake 150–300 minutes (2½–5 hours) of moderate intensity physical activity per week, with regular muscle-strengthening activity for all age groups. Studies show that 30 minutes a day has proven health and longevity benefits. Want to know how much to push yourself? Turn to page 180 for movement expert Richie Norton's recommendations. (Spoiler alert: it's not as much as you think.)

HOW

When we talk about exercise, it often feels like something that we 'have' to do, and often something we haven't got the time, inclination or energy for. But it doesn't have to mean hitting the gym at 6am and smashing a HIIT workout (hats off to you if you do that), it's more about incorporating as much movement as possible into our daily lives. And the more we move, the better we feel and sleep, so it naturally ladders up into a more active life without us having to make a huge effort.

Richie Norton is the Mind and Movement Mentor and the author of *Lift Your Vibe*. An ex professional rugby player, Richie combines his sporting background with holistic techniques including yoga, breathwork and meditation to create a really inspiring and practical approach to exercise, reframing it as something that we can all do in the here and now.

'Sleep and movement are intrinsically linked,' he says. 'I think that's the thing people don't quite grasp. We know that we need to move for our mental and physical health and it's important to keep the body challenged and healthy for as long as possible. It also directly impacts our sleep.'

What that looks like is different for everyone. 'The general fundamentals are: be less focused on what the exercise has to be and more on something that raises our heart rate, improves blood flow, gets oxygen around to the cells, maybe gets a bit of a sweat on and stimulates our body to release all those happy hormones,' Richie says. 'If we can look at where we can find those opportunities, we can get into a rhythm where we feel active, energized, focused and creative throughout our day. At the end of the day, our body is really dialled into rest and recovery, which improves the sleep depth and quality.'

Richie says that it's also important to take more of a

mind–body approach to movement and make it into a ritual that gives us purpose and meaning, rather than just something fitness-based. 'Don't overcomplicate what the activity is, as long as you're making it a form of a ritual and doing something for you. Sleep, movement, breathwork, spending time outside – they're all rituals. When we start to find a habit that makes us feel good, the more motivated and empowered we are to keep doing it.'

LOOK FOR EASY WINS

'When it comes to movement, I always say, what are the easiest, lowest hanging fruits?' says Richie. 'No matter how busy we are, we can do one thing for ourselves. It just needs to be something that causes a physical release, improves the way we breathe and provides an outlet for any stress to disperse.'

Look for easy wins in your day. 'Carry your shopping bags, go and walk up that hill. Climb up your own stairs in your house,' Richie says. If you're like me and work from home a few days a week, some days things are so crazy busy it can be hard to leave the house, let alone get to the gym. Even then, there are ways to work out. 'There's lots you can do in your home,' says Richie. 'It could be getting up and doing a few sets of bodyweight squats or lunges, or going up and down the stairs five times.' Otherwise, add some extra movement in your day. 'Even taking a meeting while you walk will get your heart rate up for those 30 minutes or less,' says Richie. 'That's what we should be focusing on, rather than what the exercise looks like. There are potential training opportunities everywhere. At the end of the day, we just have to keep moving.'

> **Top tip:** Increase the wellbeing wins by teaming your movement time with seeing others. 'If you can share it with someone, you're hitting some huge wins for social connection, de-stressing and venting, and a sense of community,' says Richie. 'All these little simple wins can eventually build up to huge health transformations.'

Movement for better sleep: Richie's top tips

* Morning time: do some energizing movement, which means anything that raises your heart rate and gives you that natural high.
* Evening time: do something relaxing and gentle that will regulate your system, especially if you've had a busy day. This could be going outside when the sun is setting and looking into low sky, rolling out your mat for a few evening stretches or a yin-based yoga routine, going for a gentle evening walk or immersion in a natural environment like your garden or balcony.
* Breathwork: for most of us, a breath exercise is the quickest way to calm the nervous system, take stress out of the body and calm the mind. The slower, deeper and smoother we can breathe, the more it will help to calm our heart rate, lower blood pressure and allow us to feel more peace. This signals to the body it's time to rest, digest and get ready for sleep.
* Consistency: just a few minutes every morning and evening will build that ritual and deepen it, because you'll soon realize how powerful it is.

RULE 7:
Do the 3-2-1 routine every night

* 3 hours before bed = no food or alcohol (water or a non-stimulating herbal tea is fine)
* 2 hours before bed = no work or strenuous exercise
* 1 hour before bed = no screens and dim the lights

WHY?

Having a regular routine of sorts makes us feel more in control of our lives, but studies have shown that it can also lower stress and anxiety and improve our connections with others. You might feel you haven't got time to put a routine in place or that it's one more thing to 'do', but that's probably a sign that you need one! A routine starts with an action, no matter how small, and can make everything else in our lives run more smoothly. As I've got older, I've really started to appreciate the importance of a dedicated evening routine. It helps me to switch off from any stresses and strife of the day and gets me into downtime mode. For me, that's lighting a candle, running a bath while I potter round the bedroom and reading a book in bed for 15–30 minutes before I turn the light off.

'We create a bedtime routine for our children, why not create one for ourselves?'
– Sleep expert Nick Witton

3 HOURS BEFORE BED = NO FOOD OR ALCOHOL

Eating 3 hours before bed is the optimum time recommended for our bodies to digest food. Eating late at night (especially if the foods are higher in carbs and sugars) stimulates our digestive system and inhibits the release of melatonin, which can interfere with our body's ability to fall asleep at a decent hour.

'In an ideal world we would aim to eat our dinner earlier than most of us do now, and then stop eating until the next morning,' says Alice Mackintosh, registered nutritional therapist and co-author of *The Happy Kitchen: Good Mood Food.* 'This allows for an overnight fast of around twelve hours and research shows that those who do this sleep better. A working digestive system can disrupt sleep and not only that, the cells of our gut are also pro-grammed to do important housekeeping at night when we sleep, which can't be done when it is digesting food. Eating earlier also gives the body time to stabilize blood sugar before bed, meaning we don't get peaks and troughs that keep us up later, or disturb sleep cycles.'

When it comes to alcohol, on average, it takes our bodies 1 hour to process one unit, with a further 2 hours to allow the alcohol to fully leave our system. Blood sugar levels are another reason why we can often have a rubbish night's sleep after having a drink. Alcohol is both a sedative and a stimulant, which is why we can crash out initially (or pass out!) only to wake up in the early hours.

'Many alcoholic drinks like wine, bubbles, cocktails or beer have added sugar in them,' says Alice. 'This wreaks havoc with our own blood sugar levels and can disturb our sleep, making us wake up early the next day.' If you ever get the white wine fear or para-noia the morning after, it could be another side effect of low blood sugar. 'When our sugar levels dip our bodies can release more cortisol as a stress response, which is another reason why we wake up early and possibly feel anxious the next day,' Alice says.

Full transparency here: I found the 3-hour rule one of the trickiest to implement. I was used to having a glass of wine at 9pm at least twice a week, either after dinner at home or if I was out seeing friends, and I would often sleep badly afterwards. Implementing this rule has made one of the biggest improvements to my sleep. It does take a bit of adjusting and thinking ahead and you do still have to allow for a bit of fun and spontaneity. Rather than cancelling social plans, think about ways to tweak them. If you're going out, suggest meeting for a drink or dinner earlier. You never know, it might suit others as well. If you've got kids, try eating a bit earlier with them. Evenings can be tricky for lots of us, so if you're struggling just try to leave as big a gap as possible between mealtimes and bed. Sometimes things don't go to plan – remember, we're aiming for progress, not perfection. If I do have the odd late dinner or drink, I just accept I'm probably not going to sleep as well that night. The positives still outweigh the benefits: I had a really nice time catching up with friends with the knowledge I can get back on track the next morning.

2 HOURS BEFORE BED = NO WORK OR EXERCISE

Strenuous exercise causes our body to release endorphins that fire up brain activity, as well as increase our core body temperature, which signals to our body clock that we need to be awake. High activity exercise later in the evening (for example, running or HIIT classes) can also disrupt our hormonal balance and stop the production of the sleep hormone melatonin, which starts to naturally rise around 2 hours before we go to sleep. Some form of movement is still important to help our bodies and brains unwind from the day though, especially if you've been sitting in one position at a desk for long periods. Try doing some gentle stretching exercises or a yin-based yoga routine instead (see Rule 6).

1 HOUR BEFORE BED = NO SCREEN TIME AND DIM THE LIGHTS

We probably know that scrolling through Facebook and Instagram, online shopping or following Twitter spats isn't always the best way to relax, but that doesn't stop us. A study found that 90 per cent of American adults regularly used some form of electronic device before bed. As well as avoiding disappearing down a social media hole for an hour, there's another good reason we should be putting our screens down and that's the blue light that is emitted by smartphones, laptops, computers, tablets, e-readers, gaming systems and TV screens.

We have light receptors in our eyes, which communicate daytime signals to our brains to stay awake, and these light receptors are especially susceptible to blue light. As we discussed earlier, natural blue light is what helps to wake us up in the morning, but studies show that too much artificial blue light in the evening suppresses the production of melatonin, the all-important ingredient for facilitating the onset of sleep.

If you can't stay off your phone (and we all have those nights), swapping to Night Shift is an option, but it might not be the silver bullet for better sleep. A study by Brigham University in the US compared the sleep outcomes of 167 people in three categories: those who used their phone at night with the Night Shift function turned on, those who used their phone at night without Night Shift and those who did not use a smartphone before bed at all. The study found no discernible difference in sleep quality for the group using Night Shift compared to those using their phone without using Night Shift mode, including the time it took to fall asleep, waking after sleep onset, sleep quality and duration of sleep. Participants who went phone free before bed showed superior sleep quality compared to both other groups. Researchers concluded that the mental engagement with phones – messaging, scrolling and using social media – was a more significant factor in affecting sleep quality than just blue light alone. So for the best chances of a good night's sleep, it's probably best to put our phones away in a drawer or leave them downstairs!

Let's talk telly

Most of us like to watch something of an evening and TVs do have less blue light than other devices. But watching TV before bedtime still isn't great for our sleep. Too much telly can lead to 'time shifting', which is a delayed bedtime and later rise time. Research by the American Academy of Sleep Medicine found that 88 per cent of American adults and 95 per cent of 18–44-year-olds have lost sleep because they stayed up to watch multiple episodes of a TV show or streaming series. Binge-watching has also been linked to poor sleep quality and insomnia, while people who watch violent or distressing content are more likely to experience disturbing dreams. So as gripping as that new crime drama is, it might not be the best thing to watch before you head off to bed.

Bedtime stories

Reading before bed is a great way to switch off and detach from screens and it's a steadfast part of my routine. I always have a pile of books by my bed and I read every night before I go to sleep, even if it's only for 15 minutes. It's an easy way for me to switch off without really having to try and transport my brain from daytime busy zone to bed zone. Although I love reading physical books, they aren't for everyone. Some people choose Kindles that emit much lower levels of blue light than a phone or tablet, and although they can be an alternative, you could try an audiobook instead and use the timer setting so that it switches off after half an hour, once you've fallen asleep.

Dim the lights

It's not just about the screens. LED lightbulbs are often seen as a more environmentally friendly option because they consume less energy and last longer, but they also emit more blue light than traditional incandescent bulbs. LED light is good for targeted light, so they're used in things like kitchen recesses, bathroom mirrors and fridges. So even if you have a 3-2-1 bedtime routine, you could be unintentionally getting little bursts of blue light just by moving around the house.

Ideally you want to start dimming switches or lowering lighting (i.e. switching from ceiling lights to lamps) 2 hours before you go to sleep. Think about where you can swap artificial light for natural light with a lower lux.

One candle is around one lux measurement, so lighting candles in the evening (where safe to do so) is the perfect way to start the descent into relaxation and sleep. Red salt lamps are also good, as the pinky-red light mimics the slower wave light found in sunrises and is another way of telling our brains it's time for bed. If you use dimmer switches, not all LED lights are dimmer compatible, so research before you buy and look for ones that are low flicker or flicker free.

While lux measures the amount of light hitting a particular surface, lumens measure the general amount of light emitted by a light source. Light bulbs are measured in lumens – the higher the lumen, the brighter the bulb, and vice versa. To dim the lights enough at nighttime, use light bulbs that are 230–250 lumens, which is the lowest level.

The 'Three good things' list

One other thing that I've started doing over the past year that really has made a difference to my bedtime routine is keeping a little notebook by my bed to keep a gratitude journal. Every night before I go to sleep, I jot down three things that went well that day. This isn't just to pat myself on the back; gratitude is actually good for us.

In the field of positive psychology, which focuses on finding what makes people thrive as opposed to what they are struggling with, there are loads of studies showing that gratitude is consistently associated with higher levels of happiness. Our brains can tend to cling on to the bad things and in my experience the time before bed is often when we can let those negative thoughts take over. A regular gratitude practice, no matter how small, can help us to build positive emotions, relish good experiences, build resilience and generally get the most out of life.

This has been another revelation in my own life, as I'm consistently amazed that even on the bad days, there's always something that makes me think: 'Wasn't that a nice moment?' It makes me go to sleep with a smile on my face, which in turn I think helps me feel less stressed. No matter how tired I am now, I always do it. It takes me no more than a minute and makes me think, 'You had three really good things happen to you and that happiness would have otherwise passed you by.' According to Suzy Reading, author of *Self-Care for Tough Times,* this is because it 'shifts you from focusing on your to-do list to the what got done list'. (See Rule 8 for Suzy's brilliant tips on rest and relaxation.)

Want to deepen your gratitude groove? Try adding a part two. 'You know what went well and what you're feeling grateful for today,' says Suzy. 'The next thing I want you to ask is: "Why did that thing happen?" Not what happened or why you're grateful it happened, but *why* did it happen? For example: "I had a really nice conversation with my mum. Why did that conversation happen?" Because we care about each other and we're well connected.' This induces what Suzy calls an 'upward spiral of joy'. 'It helps us end the day with a sense of peace: "This is what the world has brought to me and this is my part in it."'

So why not try it tonight? Take a moment to think about three good things that happened today. Write them down, no matter how small. Then ask yourself, why did they happen?

The NEOM Sleep Routine

The 3-2-1 evening routine is such a useful technique that it's become a go-to when using our products. Our approach has always been threefold: have something to inhale, something to apply and something to boost, and the Sleep Routine ticks all those boxes, with 94 per cent of people agreeing that it prepares you for a good night's sleep.* It's something I'm quite religious about incorporating into my bedtime routine, even if it's just one or two elements. It feels like a real treat at the end of the day and I know I'll sleep better that night.

* Independent blind study of one hundred volunteers over seven days using the NEOM Sleep Routine: Perfect Night's Sleep 3-wick candle, Bath Foam, Body Oil and Pillow Mist.

Step 1: Set the scene 2 hours before bedtime by lighting a Perfect Night's Sleep Candle, which is blended with a complex blend of dreamy essential oils including lavender, chamomile and patchouli, and let the scent fill the room. You could use a NEOM Wellbeing Pod and an Essential Oil blend instead – whatever you prefer – to fill the room with fragrance.

Step 2: Run a warm bath using the Perfect Night's Sleep Bath Foam. That's my go-to as I particularly like the smell of lavender, but if you're not a big lover of floral fragrances, Bedtime Hero is another great sleep blend. It's more fruity and contains chamomile, sweet ylang ylang and warming cedarwood.

Step 3: Sit in the bath for at least 10–15 minutes. This might sound quite prescriptive, but it also gives enough time for the 100% natural essential oil fragrance to fill your bathroom. During this time I might also do the 7/11 breathing technique (breathe in for 7 seconds and out for 11 seconds) at a slow and steady pace.

Step 4: Apply our Perfect Night's Sleep Body Oil on to damp skin and massage in. Start from your feet and move upwards in circular motions with long, soft strokes. Next I put on my PJs and blow out the candle. Once in bed, I spray 2–3 spritzes of the Pillow Mist, lie back and breathe deeply. Ta dah – ready for a great night's sleep!

> Why not add . . . Perfect Night's Sleep Magnesium
> Body Butter:
> Magnesium is a natural mineral that helps to calm
> the nervous system, and studies suggest that
> increasing our levels improves sleep quality.
> Containing magnesium and other skin loving
> ingredients, this gorgeously thick and luxurious butter
> provides the perfect segue into sleep.

This is the 7/11 breathing technique where you breathe in for
7 seconds and out for 11 seconds. I use it all the time, particularly in the bath after a long day. When our inhalations become

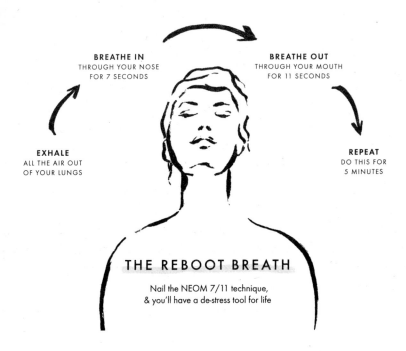

BREATHE IN
THROUGH YOUR NOSE
FOR 7 SECONDS

BREATHE OUT
THROUGH YOUR MOUTH
FOR 11 SECONDS

EXHALE
ALL THE AIR OUT
OF YOUR LUNGS

REPEAT
DO THIS FOR
5 MINUTES

THE REBOOT BREATH

Nail the NEOM 7/11 technique,
& you'll have a de-stress tool for life

longer than our exhalations, it's a sure sign of heightened stress. Inhalation stimulates the sympathetic system (accelerating heart rate and raising blood pressure) and exhalation stimulates the parasympathetic system (decreasing heart rate and lowering blood pressure). When the two branches of our nervous system are working in perfect opposition, our in and out breaths are naturally balanced. By consciously lengthening our exhalation, our heart rate slows, blood pressure drops and the muscles relax. This is a super simple and effective technique that you can use first thing, on the daily commute, or to de-stress when get home.

RULE 8:
Set aside 15 minutes for 'relaxation'
(whatever that means to you) at any point in your day

My view of relaxation has always been about creating little moments in daily life. It doesn't have to be a big or expensive gesture; it can be something in the moment that's much more achievable, like that quick soak in the bath, savouring a nice cup of tea in the afternoon, leaving your phone behind and getting outside for a bit of fresh air, or even lighting a candle while you do the ironing or put the laundry away.

We've discussed the strong link between sleep and stress, so this rule is all about giving yourself a little time out. If you're already thinking you haven't got time to relax, think of it like this: 15 minutes is approximately 1 per cent of our day. So no matter what's going on, we can all dedicate 1 per cent for some R&R time!

'Invest in rest.'

SELF CARE
is how you take your
POWER back

Suzy Reading is a chartered psychologist and NEOM's go-to self-care expert. I always describe Suzy as the most soothing hug of a person you could ever wish to meet; she is the kind of psychologist who provides a great mixture of giving you useful, new advice along with a big hug, and a little nudge forward to take action. Suzy always reframes things in a way that gives me a more well-rounded perspective on what I'm going through, which can turn around a bad day.

'We have to learn the skill of relaxation.'

Interview with the expert: Suzy Reading

Q: So Suzy, what's the link between stress and sleep?
A: Stress and sleep are intimately linked. Stress levels impact on our ability to get to sleep and the quality of our sleep. The quality of our sleep then mediates how we experience events in our waking lives. If we've poorly slept, we tend to view life through a different lens. Studies show that if we've had a bad night's sleep, we're more likely to interpret other people's facial expressions as hostile, even when they're neutral. If we've had a good night's sleep, something might feel challenging, but we feel more capable to deal with it. When we've had a rubbish night's sleep, that

same thing can potentially overwhelm us. So it's about our capacity to deal with stress. It's a dual feedback loop.

Q: How else can poor sleep affect us?
A: It affects immune function. Research shows that people who have less sleep are four times more likely to catch a cold, while poor sleep can have an impact on the hormones that regulate our appetite and feelings of fullness (see page 226 for more). When we are sleep-deprived we're not only hungrier and less satisfied by our food but it also makes us crave foods that are high in calories, fatty and carbohydrate rich.

Q: How about mentally?
A: Poor sleep can affect our consolidation of memories, cognitive performance and our concentration. It also affects our decision-making capacity: if you think about any goal that's important to you, when you're well rested, you're more able to make the decisions that support you in that goal pursuit. Sleep literally boosts our willpower.

Q: How else can it affect us?
A: It's also harder to empathize with others when we haven't slept well, and we tend to have greater feelings of anger, hostility, hypersensitivity and depression. We need good sleep, not just for our own physical and mental health, but also for the health of our relationships. Good sleep gives us the access to being kind, compassionate and empathetic individuals.

Q: This really hammers home the importance of respecting our sleep needs.
A: Absolutely. But it's important to remember that just as getting a poor night's sleep can be this downward spiral, a good night's sleep

is going to have knock-on effects in a really positive way. You don't even have to care about sleep per se. It's about what you care about in life and how sleep will enhance your ability to make that thing happen. When we reclaim our ability to rest and relax and have those little pockets throughout our day, we increase our chances of a better night's sleep and all the other benefits that come with it.

Q: A large part of it is that sometimes it's hard to know what 'relaxing' actually looks like.

A: Rest and relaxation have become synonymous with sedentary screen time. I think that's exacerbated by our experiences of the pandemic and our fatigue when it comes to social interaction and actually getting out of the house. It's also that we just don't know how to switch off. Work pervades all aspects of our life: we've got WhatsApp groups and things pinging and buzzing at us all the time. If it's not work, it's life admin, school admin, parental responsibilities. It's almost like we have forgotten how to move out of 'doing' mode back into 'being' mode. There's even a sense of striving when it comes to our downtime: we've got to prepare the perfect meal, our garden has to be perfect, our houses have to look perfect. I think a good dose of tenderness and gentleness towards ourselves would go an awful long way. Less is more.

Q: This rule is built around finding 15 minutes a day to relax. Why is it so important and how does it help us get a good night's sleep?

A: It's just so vital that we learn the skill of relaxation. The inability to relax is one of the greatest barriers to getting to sleep. If we don't know how to relax, how can we get to sleep? If we're just shoehorning these restorative practices into the 30 minutes before we go to bed, it can build pressure, e.g. 'I've got to relax now, I've got to switch off.'

> ### 'Rest and relaxation has become synonymous with sedentary screen time.'
> – Suzy Reading

Q: How do we do that?
A: We need to prioritize little soothing moments throughout the whole day to build the skill of relaxation, but also to help reduce stress levels because it has a cumulative effect. Because life keeps 'life-ing'. If we don't have an opportunity to move through the energetic charge of our emotions to just vent and let off steam, by the end of the day we're like Mount Vesuvius. You have to learn the skill of relaxation.

Q: How could rest and relaxation look to somebody who has no idea where to start?
A: It's really helpful if we can start with gentle coaxing with our inner dialogue. We can do the most gorgeous restorative practice and have a yoga session with a candle on but if we're still trash-talking to ourselves during it, or telling ourselves it's a waste of time, we fritter away the juiciness of the experience. So it's pretty fundamental that we need to cultivate kind self-talk. That's the starting point.

Q: I think people can struggle with the concept of talking kindly to themselves. Can you give some examples?
A: I give myself permission to feel. I am gentle with myself. I soften into this moment. I can give myself a break – for the next 60 seconds, the world can wait. My depletion serves no one and my replenishment serves every person my life touches.

Suzy's four tips for relaxation:

1.   **Relaxation doesn't have to mean lying down and doing nothing**. It helps to know that there are different ways in. We can use the body, for example, going for a walk because we've actually got a bit of pent-up energy that we need to let go of. It could be in the form of a gentle walk, having a stretch or doing a restorative pose like 'legs up the wall'.

2.   **Try touch**. When we extend touch or receive touch, whether that's from someone else or extending it to ourselves, we release oxytocin, which is a signal to the body to say what is safe, so that helps us relax. 'Even applying a little hand balm after you've washed your hands takes thirty seconds but it can make all the difference to how you feel.'

3.   **Honour your needs**. Sometimes we feel like we must be available around the clock, when in actual fact it would be fine if we took a 15-minute walk around the block. If we're not sleeping well, it's also important to not be tough on ourselves. Rather than berating ourselves, which only adds to our stress, acknowledge that we're having a tough time sleeping but things can change.

4.   **Be kind to yourself**. If we can be compassionate with ourselves, we can cultivate the ability to rest and adjust our expectations until we're sleeping better. It's about showing ourselves all the gentleness.

Kindness self-talk to try:

* I give myself permission to feel.
* I can be gentle with myself.
* I soften into this moment.
* I can give myself a break – for the next 60 seconds, the world can wait.
* My depletion serves no one and my replenishment serves every person my life touches.

MEDITATION

There are three other essential techniques that you will have heard a lot of hype about recently that I think are really worth setting aside time for. The first being meditation.

If you've read other books about wellbeing, you are probably aware of the benefits of meditation and mindfulness, but if you have previously thought it to be quite 'woo woo' and outdated, I think you'll be surprised at how achievable, realistic and helpful it can be. Modern meditation has moved on a lot, and you don't have to be super zen or spend hours sitting on a yoga mat to achieve a sense of inner peace. Meditative moments can be built into our day and can be as simple as slowing down a bit. You don't have to go off and 'do' meditation: even paying a bit more attention to your normal everyday tasks instead of doing them on autopilot can bring us out of our heads and back into the moment.

At a biological level, meditation has been shown to slow down the heart rate and rate of breathing. It can also help to reduce levels of rumination (those persistent thoughts that can keep us up at night) as well as calming the nervous system before sleep. Research suggests that different types of meditation can help with insomnia and even improve the sleep quality of people who don't have existing sleep problems. So a meditation or mindfulness practice, no matter how small, can add up to pretty impressive results for our sleep.

Meditation doesn't mean having to clear our minds of all thoughts, which, let's be honest, unless you're a Zen master is pretty impossible for 99 per cent of us. Suzy says, 'From my perspective, the mind is designed to think, just as the eyes are designed to see, so let's not worry about trying to stop the mind from thinking . . . The purpose of meditation is to direct the mind on to a chosen anchor. Every time that it moves away from it, without giving ourselves a tough time, we just notice and we bring it back to the anchor. It's turning an everyday activity into a meditation, and this is how we can make it accessible. It doesn't have to be an extra thing. It can be a way of doing something we're already doing.'

YOGA AND STRETCHING

The second one I think is really worth investing a bit of time in is yoga. Again, if it isn't something you do already, you might have preconceptions about it being people showing off in expensive leggings, but anyone can do it. There are endless beginner videos online (I particularly like Gaia, which has lots of free videos, and Frame, where you can book to live-stream yoga classes too) and there are so many benefits. Most importantly, it isn't just good for our waking minds and bodies – it's good for shuteye too. Moving the focus to our breath and bodies helps to calm busy minds, while gentle movement improves blood flow and releases muscle tension, all of which put us on the right side of sleep. A standard modern-day yoga practice including posture exercise, meditation and breathwork has been shown to help regulate the immune system, circadian rhythm and cardiac function, as well as increasing melatonin levels and reducing hyperarousal.

All in all, it's a convincing argument for fitting in some sort of evening restorative practice. A short routine, or even just doing a few stretches (we stretch our way into the day so why not stretch our way out of it?), is a great way to drop off the stresses and strains of the day before we head for bed, instead of taking them with us.

James Rafael is a movement and meditation coach at holistic hotel brand Equinox and is a senior teacher at Triyoga in London. I love his calm, compassionate approach, and James draws on practical techniques from the traditions of yoga, meditation and qigong (pronounced 'chi-gong'), which is an ancient Chinese medicine and philosophy practice involving the body, breath and mind. 'A short pre-bedtime stretching sequence is one of the things that has most dramatically improved my sleep over recent years,' he says. 'Combining these three poses [see pages 91–3] can give a total body and mind release to help you fall asleep faster and stay asleep longer. I'd recommend holding each pose for 1–3 minutes right before you get into bed.'

Yoga nidra

If you go to yoga classes already you may have seen a yoga nidra class at your local studio and wondered what it's all about. Essentially it is a form of guided meditation also known as 'yogic sleep'. It's become an increasingly popular tool in recent years for stress reduction, sleep efficiency and soothing our jangled nervous systems. James says: 'Yoga nidra is a powerful technique that helps you deeply relax and enter a blissful state between consciousness and sleep. The practice shifts us from the more active beta brain waves we experience in an awakened state to more restorative and mood-enhancing alpha waves.'

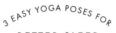

BETTER SLEEP

1. PIGEON POSE

DIFFICULTY LEVEL: BEGINNER

'So much of the tension we feel in our lower back actually originates in the deep glutes. Sitting all day and not using these powerful muscles can cause them to tighten or spasm, presenting as tension that radiates throughout the body, often without us realizing it. Pigeon gets deep into the external rotators of the hip and is a powerful tool to release whole body tension and mental stress. Beginners who are particularly tight in the pose should be careful about easing into the pose and putting too much weight on the hips.'

STEP 2
BRING YOUR RIGHT KNEE
BEHIND AND TOUCHING
YOUR RIGHT WRIST

STEP 1
START ON HANDS
AND KNEES IN A TABLE
TOP POSITION

STEP 3
GENTLY WIGGLE YOUR RIGHT
FOOT FORWARD UNTIL YOU
START TO FEEL A MODERATE
STRETCH IN THE OUTER
RIGHT HIP AND BUTT MUSCLES

STEP 8
GENTLY EXIT AND
CHANGE SIDES

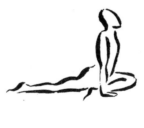

STEP 4
MINDFULLY SLIDE OR CREEP
YOUR LEFT KNEE BACK UNTIL
THE LEG IS STRAIGHT

STEP 7
FOCUS ON LONG CALM
EXHALES, AND REMAIN HERE
FOR 1–3 MINUTES

STEP 5
IF YOUR RIGHT HIP IS FLOATING
OFF THE FLOOR, PLACE A
CUSHION OR ROLLED
UP TOWEL BENEATH IT

STEP 6
LOWER ON TO YOUR FOREARMS
AND ALLOW YOUR HEAD TO
RELEASE DOWNWARDS

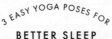

3 EASY YOGA POSES FOR

BETTER SLEEP
2. KING ARTHUR'S POSE

DIFFICULTY LEVEL: INTERMEDIATE

'Most of our lives are spent sitting, with the front of the hips in a closed/flexed position (this pattern is maintained if you are a side sleeper). King Arthur's pose dramatically stretches quads and hip flexors, which not only helps to reset this pattern, but also can positively impact your ability to breathe easily, because of the connection of the deep hip flexors (psoas muscles) around the connection of your diaphragm.'

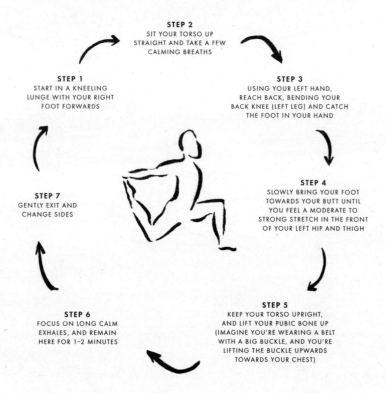

STEP 2
SIT YOUR TORSO UP STRAIGHT AND TAKE A FEW CALMING BREATHS

STEP 1
START IN A KNEELING LUNGE WITH YOUR RIGHT FOOT FORWARDS

STEP 3
USING YOUR LEFT HAND, REACH BACK, BENDING YOUR BACK KNEE (LEFT LEG) AND CATCH THE FOOT IN YOUR HAND

STEP 7
GENTLY EXIT AND CHANGE SIDES

STEP 4
SLOWLY BRING YOUR FOOT TOWARDS YOUR BUTT UNTIL YOU FEEL A MODERATE TO STRONG STRETCH IN THE FRONT OF YOUR LEFT HIP AND THIGH

STEP 6
FOCUS ON LONG CALM EXHALES, AND REMAIN HERE FOR 1–2 MINUTES

STEP 5
KEEP YOUR TORSO UPRIGHT, AND LIFT YOUR PUBIC BONE UP (IMAGINE YOU'RE WEARING A BELT WITH A BIG BUCKLE, AND YOU'RE LIFTING THE BUCKLE UPWARDS TOWARDS YOUR CHEST)

TOP TIP
If it's too intense to catch the back foot with your hand, you can use a hand towel around the foot instead and pull the foot inwards using it.

3 EASY YOGA POSES FOR

BETTER SLEEP

3. SUPPORTED FISH POSE

DIFFICULTY LEVEL: BEGINNER

'We spend a lot of our time with the upper spine in a rounded position and the chest collapsed. This pose helps to release the chest and shoulders, frees up the breath, and can have a feeling of "resetting" the whole spine.'

STEP 2
SIT DOWN WITH YOUR LEGS STRETCHED OUT IN FRONT, AND PLACE THE BOOK ON THE GROUND BEHIND YOU (ABOUT WHERE YOUR MID-UPPER BACK WOULD BE WHEN LYING DOWN, YOU WANT THE YOGA BRICK BOOK POSITIONED HORIZONTALLY, SO IT'S WIDE ACROSS YOUR UPPER BACK)

STEP 1
FIND A YOGA BRICK (OR A BIG THICK BOOK LIKE A DICTIONARY)

STEP 3
SLOWLY EASE YOURSELF DOWN, WIGGLING TO POSITION THE BRICK/BOOK RIGHT BEHIND THE CENTRE OF YOUR CHEST AND HEART, IN YOUR MID UPPER BACK

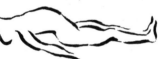

STEP 7
GENTLY EXIT THE POSITION AND LIE DOWN FLAT TO THE FLOOR AFTERWARDS TO LET YOUR BACK SETTLE AND RELAX

STEP 4
ALLOW YOUR HEAD TO RELEASE BACKWARDS TO REST ON THE FLOOR (OR A CUSHION IF IT DOESN'T COME ALL THE WAY DOWN)

STEP 6
FOCUS ON LONG CALM EXHALES, AND REMAIN HERE FOR 1–3 MINUTES

STEP 5
TAKE YOUR ARMS OUT TO THE SIDES (OR OVERHEAD) TO STRETCH YOUR WHOLE CHEST AND SHOULDER GIRDLE

Unlike a normal yoga class, yoga nidra doesn't involve any movement. Lying down in 'corpse pose', you're typically guided by a teacher or a recording through a relaxation process, using visualizations and different techniques. If you can't find or don't fancy an in-person class, a quick search online will garner an array of different free audio and video practices you can listen to at your leisure.

BREATHING TECHNIQUES

The third and final essential technique game-changer when it comes to investing in your rest is something we've already touched on: breathing. I shared the 7/11 breathing technique on page 81, which is perfect to do any time you want to slow things down and get into a relaxed state. Another that I find really useful is what's called Candle Breath. This easy breath-work technique gets its name because it mimics the movement of blowing out the candles on a cake. 'Candle breath is powerful because it releases the jaw and we hold an awful lot of tension in the jaw and the mouth,' explains Suzy. 'It also lengthens the exhalation, which is naturally calming and soothing, as well as just giving us something to focus on.'

Here's how you do it:

1.   Make sure you're sitting upright and are comfortable.

2.   Put one hand on your chest, and take a deep breath in.

3.   Imagine that there's a lit candle in front of you (a NEOM Happiness Candle is a good choice) and exhale slowly, with pursed lips.

4.   Ideally you should be aiming to make the candle flicker, rather than blowing it out.

5.   Repeat as many times as you like.

CREATE A HAVEN

My final piece of advice for how to take your downtime to the next level is this: a clean bedroom equals a serene mind. One US survey found that participants took longer to fall asleep in a messy bedroom and, unsurprisingly, felt more tired and over-whelmed the next day. That includes keeping any work or study paraphernalia out of the bedroom and especially not answering emails in bed. Another 2020 study of 2,000 people found that 84 per cent of those who'd been working from their bedroom during the pandemic found their sleeping pattern was either 'disrupted' or 'very disrupted' as a result.

RULE 9:
Make your bedroom a tech-free zone that's as dark as possible and between 16 and 19°C

WHY?

We looked at light in depth in Rule 5 (see page 61) but to reiterate, ditching all LED devices (phones, tablets, laptops) before bedtime is a must for good sleep. As well as sending an alerting effect telling our brains to stay awake, the blue light from devices can also cause a spike in our cortisol levels, which causes our hearts to beat faster and our blood pressure to rise. As I mentioned earlier, reading is a great way to relax before bed but unfortunately studies have shown that reading on an iPad suppresses melatonin levels (our sleep-friendly hormone) by up to 50 per cent, compared to a printed book. So, to sum it up: bright light at bedtime is not our friend and you're much better off swapping your tablet for a printed book or an audiobook as I mentioned earlier.

> Recent studies have found that around 75 per cent of children and 70 per cent of adults use electronic devices in their bedroom or in bed.

TURN THE TEMPERATURE DOWN

Another key factor in getting a good night's sleep is our body temperature. Our core temperature is around 37°C during the day but tends to drop towards nighttime. This signals to the body that it's time for sleep and is something that happens across all mammals. Typically, we experience a 1–2 degree drop in temperature, which starts to happen around 2 hours before sleep. During sleep our body temperature continues to fall, reaching a low point around 2–4am, before gradually warming up as we move towards waking up.

It might be tempting to whack up the heating, especially on cold nights, but like light, temperature has a big impact on sleep. Studies show that a bedroom that is too warm can interfere with our body's temperature regulation process and lead to fatigue, that frustrating scenario when we're lying in bed feeling tired but not being able to sleep. Experts say that 16–19°C is the ideal bedroom temperature, signalling to the body that it's time to wind down.

Why a hot bath really works (and not for the reason you might think)

If you're familiar with NEOM, you'll know we love a bath. It's always been a non-negotiable part of my evening routine, whatever I've been doing that day or wherever I've been. Even a quick soak feels like a proper relaxation and a bit of time to myself. And aside from the R&R factor, an evening bath has scientific benefits for sleep.

While we might think a hot bath gets us nice and warm and cosy for a good night's sleep, it actually does the opposite. As we've said, our body temperature needs to drop in order to fall asleep properly and, in fact, having a warm bath activates a process called vasodilation, which involves sending the heat away from our core and increasing the blood flow to our hands, feet and skin, where that heat gets released. Matthew Walker, neuroscientist and author of *Why We Sleep*, describes this process as 'charming the heat' out of our body.

Studies suggest that the ideal water temperature for an evening soak is 40°C and that a bath is best taken 1 to 2 hours before bedtime. Research published in *Sleep Medicine Reviews* found that a warm bath or shower could help a person fall asleep and improve sleep quality, even in the height of summer. Consciously thinking about ways to cool both ourselves and our bedroom will help with temperature regulation, and signal to our bodies that it's time to sleep.

MAKE YOUR BEDROOM AS DARK AS POSSIBLE

Even at night with the lights off, our bedrooms are seldom pitch black, in fact over 80 per cent of the world lives under light-polluted skies, while new research says that nighttime light pollution is increasing by 10 per cent a year. External sources of light include landing lights, streetlights, flashing devices or lamps and blue light still being used by others. Our eyelids are very thin and don't block out all light even when they're closed, so light can still reach our retinas, which is the back part of the eye that responds to light. Invest in blackout blinds and/or wear an eye mask to ensure that no light gets through. And remember the tips from Rule 7 about toning down your lighting in the hours before bed.

Ask me anything

Q: Weighted blankets – BS or worth the money?
A: I'm not really into weighted blankets, which are meant to apply a calming amount of pressure to the body and help with things like stress reduction and anxiety. I think people either like them or don't and I feel a bit trapped when I've got one on top of me, so they've never really worked for me. They claim to regulate body temperature, but I think we can do that ourselves, plus they're very expensive!

RULE 10:
Eat three regular meals evenly spread throughout the day

WHY?

Sticking to regular mealtimes throughout the day regulates our circadian rhythms, which in turn helps to promote better sleep. What we eat and when helps our bodies to perform their natural functions, so we perform better during the day and wind down in the evening. Erratic mealtimes and a diet that makes us feel worse rather than better throws our rhythms out of whack and can lead to a whole host of side effects including tiredness, rollercoaster sugar levels and a struggling digestive system.

'The more regular we can be with our meals, the better,' says registered nutritional therapist Alice Mackintosh. 'Skipping meals, having lunch at different times, eating dinner at 6pm one day and then 10pm the next day, or grazing all day and having frequent "carby" or sugary snacks can all throw our body off its natural circadian rhythm.'

Our meals often get shoehorned into a day of deadlines, meetings, working late and caring responsibilities, but in an ideal world we should be basing our days around our mealtimes rather than the other way round. 'Getting three regular meals a day helps your body to know what's coming, and therefore, be more likely to stay within its circadian rhythm,' Alice says. 'It's about tuning into it and having those regular routines in place. Just like you go to bed at the same time, have your meals the same.'

'The body likes consistency and being in its natural flow.'

– Alice Mackintosh, registered nutritional therapist

Studies show that all the cells in our body are primed to follow their own natural daily rhythms. Disrupting these finely tuned systems can lead to problems such as sleep issues, weight gain, low energy and digestive troubles. 'For example, the pancreas has genes that switch on during times when it should produce more enzymes to break our food down and regulate our blood sugar,' says Alice. 'The gut and its trillions of bacteria also operate a circadian rhythm that allows it to digest, absorb nutrients and remove waste. Tuning into this rhythm is especially important when it comes to sleep.' Research shows that as well as waking up and going to bed at the same time each day, sticking with set mealtimes and avoiding snacking in between can encourage this natural flow, and support a good night's sleep. 'It doesn't mean you need to stick to a strict fasting routine or go for long periods without eating, but the body likes consistency and prefers to be in its natural flow where possible,' says Alice.

SLEEP-FRIENDLY FOODS

The power of protein

'When eating for sleep, one of the most important things to keep in mind is making sure that you supply your body with the right building blocks to make melatonin, the hormone that helps to bring on the onset of sleep,' says Alice. Protein is key because it provides those building blocks, so ideally you'd get some protein at every meal. 'Turkey, chicken and walnuts are especially good because they contain tryptophan, an amino acid that converts to melatonin in the brain, however it's generally a good idea to eat an array of different protein sources each day from a variety of sources,' says Alice.

Crucially, our bodies can't make tryptophan by themselves, so we need to get it from food sources. Animal-derived foods tend to contain the highest levels of tryptophan, but we can boost our sleep in other ways. Other foods that help boost melatonin levels include oats, bananas, seeds and nuts. Lots of granola brands and other so-called 'healthy' breakfast cereals can actually contain a ton of hidden sugar, so try making your own hearty bircher muesli or homemade porridge in the winter.

TRYPTO-FRIENDLY FOODS

Animal-based	Plant-based
Turkey	Tofu
Chicken	Oats/oatmeal
Salmon	Pineapple
Beans	Pumpkin and sesame seeds
Eggs	Walnuts
Milk	Butternut squash seeds
Greek yogurt	Cashews
	Peanut butter

A helping hand(ful)

Want to supercharge your day and give your sleep the best chance? Add a handful of nuts or seeds to your breakfast. 'Protein also helps to keep our blood sugar levels stable,' says Alice. 'So if we make a bowl of porridge with oats, banana and honey, it's good for us in lots of respects, but there's not really any protein in that meal. If you were to add a handful of seeds or nuts, you end up with less of a spike in your blood sugar, and more of a sort of gentle rise.' This gives way more stabilized blood sugar levels over the day and through the night, which is very important for sleep. 'Adding a handful of nuts also turbocharges the vitamins and minerals, so it's a real secret weapon,' Alice says.

Magnesium

'Eating plenty of magnesium-rich foods in the diet is vital, because this mineral is also important for helping to make melatonin,' says Alice. 'Magnesium helps to induce the release of GABA, another calming brain chemical that we release in the lead up to sleep. Magnesium-friendly foods also relax our muscles and nervous system, which helps us feel calm and ready for sleep.'

Look for magnesium in green leafy veg like pak choi, kale, spinach and broccoli, as well as in whole grains (rice, quinoa, pasta) and nuts and seeds like cashews, almonds, pumpkin seeds and peanuts. 'Raw cacao and 70+ per cent dark chocolate are also a great source,' says Alice. 'Try to have them earlier in the day as both contain caffeine and a plant molecule called theobromine which can also energize you.'

B vitamins

If you want a good night's sleep, it's vital to load up on the B vits. 'B vitamins are absolutely critical [to good sleep] and a deficiency negatively affects many body systems,' says Alice. 'They also help us cope better with stress and help with thyroid and female hormone balance, which can also impact our sleep cycles, especially in perimenopausal women where sleep can be profoundly disturbed.'

There are eight kinds of B vitamins, which are found in a variety of foods including meat, fish, seafood, lentils, beans, whole grains and vegetables like avocado, beetroot and sweet potatoes. 'If you're vegan, it's a good idea to get your B12 levels checked yearly because B12 is only found in animal sources of food like meat, eggs and dairy,' adds Alice.

'B vitamins are absolutely critical to good sleep.'

– Alice Mackintosh

The F word

'Put simply, think of the three Fs: fibre, fermented foods and (healthy) fats,' says Alice. 'All of these work to support our microbiome, reduce inflammation and support the complex network that exists between our brain and our gut (you can read more about gut health on page 134). 'Though eating foods to support your gut won't necessarily lead to you feeling sleepy right there and then, it can contribute towards better mood, brain health and stress management, all of which positively impact our ability to sleep well.'

The three Fs:

1.   Fibre = whole grains, beans, lentils, colourful vegetables, fruit, nuts, seeds

2.   Fermented foods = kimchi, kombucha, kefir, sauerkraut and other pickled veggies

3.   Fat = oily fish (especially mackerel and anchovies), avocado, almonds, walnuts, flaxseeds, extra virgin olive oil.

Alice's other sleep-friendly staples:

1.   All **nuts** are really nutritious, but things like walnuts, pistachios, almonds and Brazil nuts are really good. Two palmfuls a day is a good amount. I like to add them to porridge but you can also roast them, or sprinkle them over salads. **Nut butters** like almond butter and peanut butter are also good. Choose ones that don't have any other added ingredients, so no palm oil and no sugar.

2. **Seeds** – hemp seed in particular is rich in sleep-supporting nutrients, as is flaxseed (the former should be kept in the fridge for freshness).

3. **Tahini** is very nutritious and is basically made up of sesame seeds. It's a very versatile ingredient; you can put it into porridge (you'd need to put a bit of sweetener like fruit in there as well), use it in salad dressings or blend it into a lot of healthy baking.

4. **Fish** contains omega 3, which is very important for our brain and in particular anxiety and mood. Any fresh fish is good but oily fish like smoked salmon or mackerel pate are good options.

5. **Whole grains**, so brown rice, quinoa, oats, anything you fancy, but not white grains as they spike your blood sugar levels, plus whole grains contain more fibre and nutrients than white grains. **Whole grain pasta** and **spelt pasta** are also good options.

6. **Beans or lentils,** so things like black beans, chick-peas, red or puy lentils. You can buy them pre-cooked in pouches or tins which will save time.

7. **Herbs and spices.** Fresh herbs and spices are great; turmeric in particular has been shown to help support mental wellbeing. Cinnamon and nutmeg are also very good for mood, while saffron is particularly good for anxiety, but it's very expensive, so may be one to use sparingly.

> **Alice's top tip:** Nuts can go rancid after a few months, so keep them in the fridge for freshness. Always use in-date spices, rather than turmeric that's been in the cupboard for three years or kept near the oven!

Ideal mealtimes
* Breakfast 8–9am
* Lunch 1–2pm
* Dinner 7–8pm

'Obviously people's mealtimes differ and this isn't going to work for someone who does shift work,' Alice says. 'Some like to wait till 10am to eat their breakfast while others might eat with their kids. It really depends on what suits you, but ideally you won't have eaten for at least 12 hours before you have breakfast and it's best not to eat between meals to avoid spiking your blood sugar levels. Have an afternoon snack if you feel that you need one, but leaving a gap of 4 to 5 hours helps your body do the important housekeeping it needs to do between meals. Having protein at every meal will help you feel fuller for longer, so you shouldn't feel hungry in between.'

Ask me anything

Q: I always struggle to sleep well on holiday. What's your advice?
A: It can have a lot to do with temperature control, which is obviously going to be trickier if you're in a hot country, but the one thing that throws my sleep out the most when I'm away is my routine being out of check, especially when it comes to eating later. So I try and instil as much routine as possible by reading

before bed, using the Pillow Mist and sometimes I'll even take a shower before I go to bed using Perfect Night's Sleep products. These familiar scents and behaviours remind me of my sleep routine back at home and having that continuity helps.

RULE 11:
Have your last coffee
(or caffeinated drink) by midday

I have a cup of tea in bed in the morning and a cup of good ground coffee before I leave the house, another coffee when I get to work and perhaps another somewhere before midday. On the very rare occasion, I might have a cup of tea at 4 o'clock if I felt incredibly sleepy but that's it. So I do go pretty hard on caffeine but I always do it early.

Lots of us look forward to that first coffee in the morning or a mid-morning tea break. Aside from the ritual, taste and social aspects, there are proven scientific benefits to caffeine and how it can enhance our daytime functioning. 'A little bit of caffeine has been shown to be supportive of mood, focus, energy and our general longevity,' says nutritional therapist Alice Mackintosh. 'Although more research is needed, there are some studies that show that those of us who consume a cup of coffee daily have a better chance of living longer.'

Moderation is key here and too much caffeine can be a bad thing. 'Sleep is an area where there is clear research about caffeine impacting us negatively,' says Alice. 'Caffeine in any form, e.g. tea, coffee, fizzy drinks, has a number of physiological impacts, namely on our adrenaline and cortisol. It raises the level of these two hormones, making us feel alert, energized, warm and awake.'

When caffeine becomes bad for us is when it starts to inter-fere with our sleep. 'The main thing to note when it comes to sleep and caffeine is that cortisol and adrenaline wake us up in the morning, while melatonin does the opposite in the evening,' says Alice. 'Triggering too much cortisol can disrupt our natural circadian rhythms.'

THE (SECRET) HALF-LIFE OF CAFFEINE

'Half-life' is the metric used to describe the amount of time it takes for the quantity of a substance to be reduced to half its original amount. When we drink caffeine, we can experience the effects immediately, but it has a half-life of 5 to 6 hours, which means even after that caffeine hit has worn off, it takes around 10 hours to exit our bodies completely. 'This means that half the caffeine in a cup of coffee drunk at midday will still be in your bloodstream at 5 or 6pm, but this will vary from person to person,' says Alice. 'Many people say that caffeine doesn't impact their sleep, but they may find they naturally wake up early and can't get back to sleep.' Even when we are asleep, Alice says, the body's cycles of deep sleep and REM sleep can be disrupted by caffeine, meaning we don't wake up feeling fully rested and restored.

HOW TO DO IT

Mornings can go past in a rush and we can find ourselves auto-matically reaching for another coffee, especially if it's based around an event like meeting a friend, or a work meeting. Try setting a reminder on your phone to let you know the caffeine cut-off is coming. Just having that little nudge every day should be enough to keep you on track. If you really can't do without something later, or look forward to that mid-afternoon cuppa, opt for the decaffeinated option or a herbal tea instead. Most herbal teas are 100 per cent caffeine free but matcha and green tea still contain caffeine. 'Ideally we should be aiming to limit our caffeine intake to 1–2 cups of caffeinated drinks per day and stopping after midday,' says Alice. (Note to self.)

THE GREAT CAFFEINE MYTH

Did you know that caffeine doesn't actually give us a buzz, it just stops us feeling tired? Adenosine is a neurotransmitter that promotes our sleep drive, or our need to sleep. Caffeine molecules are the same size as adenosine molecules and the way caffeine works is that the molecules bind to and block the sleep-making adenosine molecules. This stops us feeling tired, even if we really are. Eventually the caffeine molecules unbind from the adenosine receptors, allowing adenosine molecules to flood back in. This causes us to suddenly become tired, which in turn can see us reaching for another coffee. Interesting!

HORMONES AND SLEEP

As we've seen in this chapter, there are lots of things that have material impact when it comes to sleep, but taking control of our hormones isn't so easy. Many of us have probably experienced on some level a hormone-related sleep issue, whether it's sleeping a bit worse when our period is due to experiencing anxiety and nighttime hot flushes during the menopause.

Oestrogen rises during the first half of the menstrual cycle and drops during the second half, prior to menstruation. This is especially important when it comes to sleep. Professor Annice Mukherjee aka @the.hormone.doc is a medical hormone specialist and author of *The Complete Guide to the Menopause*. She says:

'Oestrogen is a feel-good hormone so if your oestrogen is low, it can impact on your sleep. It's different for every woman but you may feel more anxious, especially if you experience a sudden drop before your period. The natural progesterone our bodies produce has a calming effect, so if you've got good hormone balance your sleep shouldn't be impacted. But for many women it is a problem and things like diet, misaligned body clocks and lifestyle choices all make hormone imbalances worse. It can be a bit of a chicken and egg scenario.'

Oestrogen levels also drop during the menopause transition, which is when many women experience sleep problems. 'We tend to get what are called the "vasomotor symptoms" associated with the menopause, which can cause a change in blood supply to the skin and a change in temperature,' says Professor Mukherjee. 'These manifest as hot flushes, sweating, palpitations, feeling wide awake or maybe even a panic attack if someone has underlying stress, which can exacerbate symptoms.'

Will going on the pill help?

Some birth control pills contain high levels of oestrogen, while HRT is the most popular choice in menopause, but Professor Mukherjee says it's not as simple as that. 'Women who go on high-dose contraceptive pills don't always report positive impact on their sleep. I also see many women postmenopausal who sleep great, but people who've never slept well in their entire adult life may well experience problems in the menopause transition, because it's going to have more of a heightened effect. Our sleep and sleep rhythms are impacted by many other things. It's very multifaceted.'

FINAL THOUGHTS

Perhaps the greatest learning for me personally is that better sleep is something I can have a substantial amount of control over. It's not a predestined state, there are (lots) of real-life things I can do to improve it. Sure, some are harder for me (I'm still struggling with that no wine or food 3 hours before bed if I'm being honest, as I'm often out or having friends over and I'm a total foodie!) but at least I know *why* I've slept poorly if I do, and I'm not panicking about it. It's something I can pick up the next night.

Understanding the basics of my body clock and respecting how my circadian rhythm works is key and has been game-changing for me. Everything makes sense now and the ramifications of modern life (which for me is early meetings indoors and late-night Instagram scrolling) are clear. I've learned to be more aware of how that impacts me and have found work-arounds for getting too little light in the morning or too much at night by adjusting my routines and eating times wherever possible. In short, I DO have more control on my sleep than I thought and even just knowing that is empowering.

2.
STRESS

WHAT IS STRESS?

I've long had a fascination with stress since experiencing burn-out many years ago and it was one of the things that inspired me to start NEOM. Since then, I've made it my mission to understand modern stress, to create the best products we can and provide the best wellbeing advice for today's person experiencing stress. It's why so many of us end up feeling like we do: exhausted, anxious and overwhelmed with the feeling we haven't got the time or the answers to put things right. And yet it doesn't have to be that way.

My stress wake-up call happened back in the early noughties and since then we've only got more stressed. Rising numbers of people are reporting work-related stress and burnout, while a UK survey carried out by the Mental Health Foundation and YouGov revealed that 74 per cent of respondents said they've felt stressed to the point of feeling that they couldn't cope.

Not everyone faces chronic levels of stress on a daily basis, but most of us have felt stress impact on our lives, even in the smallest of ways. I've heard so many stress stories over the past two decades and what I've learned is that stress can look different to each of us. It can be through a lack of sleep, or our workload, family life, or just not feeling in control of things.

When it comes to stress, prevention is the number one focus. The key is to keep your absolute basics topped up every day, so your stress levels don't overflow. Just like keeping on top of my sleep, it's putting the small things in place that work (most of the time) for me. Calmness is within our control, far more than we realize, and there are often lots of simple things we can do to bring a sense of equilibrium, peace and confidence back into our lives.

'Prevention is the fundamental rule when it comes to stress.'

We can't get away from stress. It's a by-product of life. Unfortunately, it isn't something we only experience during big events like losing a job or going through a divorce, or someone we love falling ill, or living through a natural disaster. It can be the smaller things that just build up over time. Modern life by its very nature can be really stressful, and it's important to acknowledge that. Given that we can't get away from stress, it's imperative that we build up a toolkit that then helps us prevent it from becoming too big. I've come to realize over the years that when you've reached the point where stress is really bad, it's always harder to roll back from it. It's much better to start stress-proofing your life way in advance, than starting from a point of complete burnout.

One of the best stress busters I know is NEOM's self-care expert Suzy Reading. 'Stress manifests on all levels, but how that happens depends on each individual,' Suzy says. 'We've become so skilled at overriding our stress symptoms because that's what life tells us to do. It's so important to have little pauses in the day, not just for managing stress but as a chance to check in and just notice where we're at and take some kind, restorative action.'

HOW STRESSED ARE YOU?

Sometimes we don't even realize that we are stressed, particularly if we've been operating in that state for a period of time. Awareness around stress is key: just pausing to check in and see how we're feeling can be a bit of a light-bulb moment and helps us to address our stress, whether it's an immediate solution (like cancelling that thing in your diary you don't want to do) or making bigger lifestyle changes in the long term. 'Stress can show up in so many different ways,' says Suzy. 'Reflect on these questions to get to know your early warning signs and get a handle on stress. How does stress show up for you?'

Suzy Reading's stress test:

1.   Does it show up in your **thinking**, whether that's over-thinking, ruminating, worrying, catastrophic thoughts, or negative thinking?

2.   Do you feel stress in your **emotions**? That may be feeling irritable, teary, or it could be feeling distanced from our emotions, a sense of numbing.

3.   Is it reflected in your **immune system**? Do you tend to get everything that's going around, one thing after another, or have ailments that tend to linger?

4.   Do you notice stress in your **digestive health**? It can manifest in stomach upsets, constipation or it could be tension in your stomach.

5. How does stress show up in your **sleep**? Perhaps it's hard to get to sleep, get back to sleep, or you experience early morning wake-ups. Or maybe you sleep like a log and but still wake up not feeling refreshed.

6. Check in with your **physical body**: does it present as aches, pains, muscular tension, joint inflammation or headaches?

I find this list super helpful and something that I'll go back to. Take a moment to look through the list. Where does stress show up for you, and what steps can you take to remedy it?

For me, the most common one is the first one on the list, as stress typically shows up in my thought patterns. This means overthinking on little things that someone else wouldn't think twice about, or going round in circles about a certain situation with seemingly no end or answer in sight. Then I realize that I'm stressed and that's the time I need to step back. That could be going out for a walk to clear my mind, clearing my diary of anything non-essential for that day or week, or phoning/meeting a friend. I also hold stress in my body and I'll notice if my shoulders and neck are tight, or I'm sitting in the chair holding my breath. These are exactly the kind of moments that brought our products into life, so I might put on our Calming Hand Balm, which is infused with soothing lavender, jasmine and sandalwood, and do a few rounds of breathing. Otherwise, I absolutely love our Calming Pen, which is also from our Scent to De-stress range. I keep one in my handbag at all times; it's great for a moment of calm on the go. Pop it on your temples or wrists whenever you need a little self-soothing moment.

THE FOUNDATION FOR A FULL LIFE

If we don't have tools and habits that keep stress at bay, it can keep us small, anxious and doubting ourselves. Twenty years on from that burnt-out twenty-something who was working and partying too much and not looking after herself, I'm a busy working mum with a 100-strong team and a business that is constantly evolving and growing. I have to make a lot of decisions on most days, and juggle responsibility with the constant change and uncertainty that comes with running a business. On paper, I should theoretically be more stressed than ever, but over time, and with a *lot* of trial and error, I'm able to take on the challenges and actually enjoy and feel energized by them (most of the time). When you've got a much sturdier springboard to manage your stress, you're able to squeeze the juice out of life and really enjoy it.

We also shouldn't fear stress. Most of us are going to experience it, so we need to be teaching ourselves, our children and our team at work that a) it's part of life and b) we need a toolkit to make sure that we've got our own protection to deal with it. Having the right mindset, and remembering that the hard times will pass, is another huge part. It's about having a degree of acceptance that life goes through its ups and downs and you've got to ride those waves, as much as it is having a physical toolkit that works on nourishing your mind and body.

Culturally, I think part of the problem is the way in which people seem to wear stress as a badge of honour. It's something I probably noticed more in my old job, where people climbed up the career ladder and viewed things more competitively. I think that idea of success and how we work well is moving on though, and we don't have that culture at NEOM, but when you talk to friends it can still be a bit of a tit-for-tat list about all the things on our to-do lists. The entrepreneur hustle where you work every day and night doesn't have to be the norm. Don't get me wrong, you're not going to achieve your goals without good old determination and effort. But we cannot sacrifice the fuel we put in, which ultimately is our own wellbeing. What I learned first-hand – and what I attribute the success of NEOM to – is that you actually get further in life by understanding your wellbeing needs and honouring and replenishing them. This is especially important post-pandemic, when many of us suffered with some level of fatigue or burnout.

WOMEN AND STRESS

It might not come as a surprise to many of you, but the statistics show that women suffer more with stress – and its subsequent health effects. Not only that, stress has been linked as a trigger for autoimmune diseases, with women making up approximately 80 per cent of diagnosed cases. In his book *When the Body Says No*, psychologist Gabor Maté writes about how women become the 'emotional stress absorbers of their environment' and take on the stresses of everyone around them. Many of us can relate to that, and the stress we absorb as a by-product of our lives can become so entrenched that it starts to feel normal; as if we wouldn't be good mums, partners, colleagues or friends if we weren't rushing from A to B trying to fit everything and everyone else in. As with lots of things, sometimes it takes other people to point out our stress to us. I think there's a permission thing around it we often don't want to 'admit' that we've just got too much on our plate and are struggling, because that might mean we are failing in life, and so many of us strive to be all things

MY GO-TO
STRESS TOOLKIT

NUMBER ONE IS SLEEP

MICRO MOVEMENTS

NOURISHING MY BODY

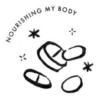

FEEDING MY MIND

CONNECTION WITH THE RIGHT PEOPLE

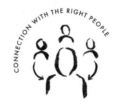

A DEGREE OF GIVING BACK

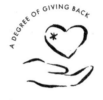

CREATIVITY

TALK TO YOURSELF AS IF YOU WERE A CHILD

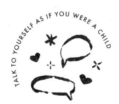

LEARNING HOW TO SAY A HIGH-QUALITY NO

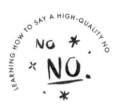

A STRESS-FREE NIGHT IN

to all people and keep those plates spinning, right? So if you are feeling stressed or overwhelmed right now, there's nothing to feel guilty or ashamed about. The best thing you can do is stop, take a breath, acknowledge where you are, tell trusted others how you're feeling and start to put a toolkit in place. Stress *is* a part of being human but when it's left unchecked, or we come to view it as a normal state of being, it can start to materially, physically and emotionally impact our lives and those around us.

THE 10 THINGS IN MY TOOLKIT

This changes over time and depends on what's going on in my life, so use these as inspiration for your own toolkit, but remember to make it achievable and personal to you.

1. A good night's sleep
Without it, everything goes out the window. It's literally the foundation of everything. I know if I prioritize my sleep and put things in place to sleep well, everything else will ladder up from that.

2. Getting outside for a walk
There's a huge body of research now on how exercise and movement help to reduce mental and physical stress. I'm not really the kind of person who goes for a run to blow away the cobwebs, so for me, it's generally getting outside for a walk.

3. Nice nourishment
This means the nourishment of my body with the right vitamins, minerals and whole foods. I'm a big fan of

science-backed natural supplements. I don't take supplements for supplement's sake and only take certain ones (like Vitamin D and B12) that I really believe in and from brands that I rate.

4. Feeding my mind with good things
I like feeding my mind with ways of looking at things that are positive yet also realistic. For example, I love the author Brianna Wiest, who wrote *101 Essays That Will Change the Way You Think*. I find her Instagram posts really inspiring and they often give me just what I need at that time.

5. Connection with the right people
Having healthy positive relationships with the right people who meet you where you are at without judgement is really important; that goes for our personal and professional lives.

6. A degree of giving back
I think generosity is a really underrated part of our toolkit and a crucial ingredient for good mental health. Research has shown that altruistic behaviour releases endorphins in the brain, which produce a positive feeling known as a 'helper's high', while other studies have linked generosity to better health. Giving back doesn't have to be a grand gesture or something formal, it could just be donating money, supporting your local foodbank or checking in with friends and family or the people you work with.

7. Some form of creativity
You don't have to be a 'creative' person to engage with creativity: it might be spending time doodling, baking or

sewing, or it might be completing a new project at work, organizing an event or visiting an inspiring new place. Creativity is also great for mental health and studies show that engaging in a creative pursuit can help to focus the mind and reduce stress and anxiety.

8. Cutting myself some slack

Self-compassion is a big one now and a lot of experts say we should talk to ourselves the way we would with our own children, or our younger selves. My own tone of voice to myself is kind, but also real, which I think I have learned to do much better as I have gotten older. I whole-heartedly believe in going easy on ourselves, but I also think we're doing ourselves a disservice if we're not being real. Self-kindness is really important if you're in a bad place for a day, or a week, or a year, or whatever it might be, but I believe that we need to pair that with being truthful and honest with ourselves and giving ourselves a firm word if needed, like we'd do with a great friend. Getting a grasp on the degree of softness that we want to take and the allowance that we want to afford ourselves is really useful. Aim for somewhere between the two: kindness along with accountability.

9. Learning how to say a high-quality no

There is so much choice in our modern society along with the pressure to keep up, be sociable and have a full life, which means we can say yes to too many things, often at our own expense. A crucial tool that everyone can benefit from, particularly the people-pleasers among us, is being fastidious about saying no to things that don't serve us, or that we can't commit to. Saying no doesn't make us selfish. It's not just saying no, but *how* we say it. The author Eckhart Tolle talks about the difference between a low- and a high-quality no: the difference being that the former comes from a place of reactivity, while a high-quality 'no' is a simple statement (for example, 'Thank you but I'm going to say no to that'). We don't have to justify or over explain our reason, it's just about saying no nicely and firmly and setting a precedent for ourselves (and others) going forward. Get comfortable saying 'no' without any guilt or shame. It can be such a simple game-changer and a great way to get stuff off your plate.

10. A stress-free night in
Netflix and a duvet, lighting a NEOM Real Luxury candle, phone switched off or in the other room, being in the company of someone I love, good food, a glass of wine and an early bath. Because, even though I have absorbed so much on wellbeing – the tips, the tricks and the latest research – sometimes the simplest things are the most nourishing for the soul. Having this in my toolkit is meaningful because when all else fails, I know that even having one night in to myself can be the reset I need; it's the one go-to I can always go to. We can say no and put ourselves first, even if it means cancelling or rescheduling plans.

Repeat after me:
My capability is not my capacity.
My free time is not my availability.
I have permission to choose.
@suzyreading

Ask me anything

Q: Cold water immersion and ice baths keep popping up on my social feed. Have you tried and do you think it's worth trying out as a de-stressing method?
A: I think cold water immersion is fantastic. It really does work and there's a lot of science about how it can help you get control over your body and brain, in terms of learning to regulate your breathing and your stress response system. Although I'm not hardcore enough to throw myself into an icy lake, turning the water to cold at the end of a shower for as long as I can works for me!

OTHER WAYS TO REDUCE STRESS

MINDFUL ACTIVITIES

I have to be honest: although I know it really works and I advised you to try it in the last chapter, I'm actually pretty rubbish at meditating. Finding some calm is essential for staying on top of stress but I think we can tweak how we do that, rather than having to find another hour on top of everything else to sit down and meditate. Whether it's having a hobby, walking the dog or listening to a podcast, there are things that we can do to bring that meditative quality to our day. For me, it's always about where I can double up on something and make it more mindful. I think that can be a really helpful way of looking at it.

Where can you double up on something and bring some still time into your day? Examples could include sitting down to savour your morning coffee instead of drinking it on the go, eating your lunch in a quiet spot away from your desk or swapping social media for a good book in your lunch hour.

MEET HARRY POTTER

Interaction with animals has been shown to lower levels of the stress hormone cortisol, and just being around animals is a great tonic for the soul. We've got loads of dogs in the NEOM office and my Westie Harry Potter is a regular on my Instagram. I'm probably the only person under eighty in my town in Yorkshire who has a Westie and I love him so much. He's just the right side of cantankerous, which you'd expect from a Westie, and quite happy doing his own thing. I have to be realistic though; I haven't got time for long walks daily, but me and H Potter just go for a little pootle around. Similarly, he'll come in the car with me and I take him along to meetings. We've had him in the office ever since he was a puppy. He's very undemanding and easy company, which is just what I need. It's very hard to feel stressed around him.

NO MORE 'ME TIME'

This might shock you, but we've banned the term 'me time' in the NEOM office. There's still this outdated view from the nineties that wellbeing is about taking a whole day or weekend to go to a spa and spend a fortune on yourself, but that's exactly what we want to get away from: the notion of having time to ourselves as this big one-off occasion that takes a lot of planning, time and money. We shouldn't feel like we've had to earn the privilege to look after ourselves. My personal view is that the phrase 'me time' still has old-fashioned connotations: that we're being selfish or self-indulgent, when actually we should be thinking of ourselves at all times, alongside everything else. I want to make wellbeing more practical and interwoven into our everyday. It's a necessity, not a luxury.

> **'The phrase "me time" has old-fashioned connotations that we're being selfish or self-indulgent, when actually we should be thinking of ourselves at all times.'**

That's not to say a lovely spa day with friends isn't something we shouldn't enjoy and look forward to, but it shouldn't be confused with basic self-care. It's taking a more informed approach to what supports your mental and physical wellbeing, not something you switch on and off, but is just pulsed into your day in very easy, manageable ways. Having a coffee and going for a walk around the block isn't 'me time', it should just be part of your routine, if that's what makes you tick. The minute you start labelling it, by inference you're saying it's selfish, so you won't do it. This is not our mission when it comes to wellbeing. I don't think it should even have a label; it's just looking after your health. You're just thinking about life in the right way.

80/20

Like everything in this book, I live by the 80/20 rule– by which I mean, make sure you've got things in place for your wellbeing 80 per cent of the time and allow the other 20 per cent to slide sometimes. There will be days where you're a bit hungover, or work's super busy, or you're running around after other people. But in my experience, once it starts getting down to 60 per cent or below is when the wheels really start to fall off. Even on the most manic days I will try to have some time to myself: whether it's listening to an interesting podcast that makes me think a bit differently on the train, or walking Harry Potter around the park for half an hour before the day starts, or stopping to get a coffee on the way back from the school run and drinking it on the park bench instead of on the run. That's proper low-level stuff for me, even if it's for 15 minutes. Even if that's my only time-out, it helps with my mindset and sets me up to stress-proof the day.

The principles of NEOM work in much the same way. It's about making your bath or shower work a bit harder for you with a really lovely, naturally fragranced product that's going to relax you or give you that boost of energy. Or else you can sit down and watch TV and have a candle packed with essential oils burning and working its magic. It's rare I would carve out a whole hour to do a self-care routine. It's more about making those moments in the everyday work a bit harder for you.

A NEOM de-stress night in

Reinvent your evening into a wellness ritual.

1.   Light a Real Luxury Intensive Skin Treatment Candle. As mentioned before, this was the first ever fragrance I created specifically for my own anxiety. It contains an elegantly complex blend of essential oils, including lavender, jasmine and sandalwood, which are all known for their super soothing, comforting properties.

2.   Run a bath and add NEOM's Real Luxury Bath Foam. Leave your phone at the door, soak for 30 minutes and feel the tension lift.

3.   Blow out the candle and allow the wax to melt and pool before pouring on the skin. Drizzle the precious oils of almond, baobab and jojoba all over the body. Massage deeply to intensively nourish and hydrate skin.

4.   Feel 'ahhh'.

'THE BRAIN CANNOT DISTINGUISH BETWEEN PHYSICAL AND EMOTIONAL PAIN'

Dr Deepak Ravindran is author of *The Pain-Free Mindset* and an expert on the nature of stress. An NHS consultant with over two decades of experience, Dr Ravindran combines a holistic approach to stress with his medical expertise in a way that makes it accessible for everyone. Stress is such a big part of our lives now and when it comes to really nailing our wellbeing, I think it's key to know the 'why' as well as the 'how'.

Interview with the expert: Dr Deepak Ravindran

Q: What's the role of cortisol in stress? It's a word that gets bandied around a lot now, but I think there's still a bit of mystery about how it all works.

A: Cortisol is a hormone that gets released by our adrenal glands, which are very tiny glands that sit on top of our kidneys. They form part of an axis, which we call the HPA or hypothalamus pituitary adrenal axis.

Q: Can you explain it in a way that's easy for people to get their heads round?

A: Think of it as a triangle: the adrenal glands are the downstream organs that respond to instructions from the pituitary gland, which is another gland in our brain. The pituitary gland itself gets its responses from an area of the brain called the hypothalamus. This hypothalamus or the 'master control' is the one that responds to stress when we perceive a threat. That threat can come from anywhere – it can be internal, meaning from within your body, so your internal organs or your gut. Or it can be external and in your environment, so your skin, emotional stresses or actual physical danger. The hormones and chemicals released from the adrenals provide a feedback loop to the hypothalamus, thus completing the triangle.

Q: So stress is a multisensory reaction?

A: Yes. And all that information is relayed from the nervous system, the hypothalamus and other parts of the brain and they make the decision on the context of the stress. Exercise puts a certain amount of stress on the body but it's a short-lived thing. If you're playing sport and you see people coming close to you, for example, that stress will be different from seeing a sabre-toothed tiger running towards you in order to harm you.

Q: Do different types of stress impact us differently?

A: Research now shows that our brain doesn't distinguish between physical and emotional pain. Whether you experience emotional stress, e.g. shock, feeling isolated, bullied, excluded or neglected; or physical stress, for example where you've sustained injuries in a road traffic accident, had a surgery, severe infection, nerve damage or any other physical pain, the part of the brain that brings these two information pieces together and decides how to protect you is the same.

Q: Where does cortisol come in?
A: A cortisol response does a variety of things. It mobilizes sugar to enter into the circulation, because we need rapid energy. It ensures that the body feels wired up and gives a rush of us 'getting ready'. It releases hormones like adrenaline, which brings about the effect of getting our hearts pumping, blood flow increasing to our muscles and more rapid breathing. It has an impact on the entire system and is preparing the body to deal with that stress, essentially as a safe measure and in a protective fashion. It becomes a bad thing when it keeps happening again and again. When that master control, the hypothalamus, is constantly releasing information that says 'release cortisol, release adrenaline, there's danger, there's stress', this amount of release is not sustainable. That's when the muscles stay constantly tight and that slips into pain. Our breathing becomes more and more rapid, until it almost feels like anxiety. As the cortisol depletes, it impacts on the immune system. We don't have the necessary response to protect us from bugs, viruses or anything going round at the time.

Q: Can we talk about the link between dopamine and stress?
A: Dopamine is the pleasure and reward chemical that produces a feel-good response in our brain. The right amount of dopamine is good for things like our learning and motivation. The downside of dopamine is that it can become an addictive cycle, which

is what people talk about with smartphone addiction, or Netflix bingeing, or anything related to social media. It's now well understood that people have small bursts of dopamine release each time they notice something that's happening, and a notification or a ping achieves that. When you're getting all these different notifications at different times, more and more dopamine keeps getting released. The more dopamine that gets released, the more it activates the release of more adrenaline and cortisol. When you are told consistently that something is about to happen, your dopamine levels actually reduce.

Q: So the surprise element you talk about keeps us in a state of low-level stress? We don't know what is coming next.
A: Exactly. Studies have found that the body releases more dopamine when we get surprised. Another example is news alerts on your phone, because the news is very varied. It can be good or bad for our brains. We don't know what the news is going to be, and so it causes a slightly higher amount of dopamine release when we open it. I think we're in the grey area of whether you call this an addictive behaviour, because we can't help opening every news feed or notification that comes along. In my view it's a minefield on how all these notifications are taking advantage and hacking our brain chemicals. There's a big digital media education drive in schools to protect our children and switch off notifications and have clearly defined periods of the day where they engage with social media, to prevent their dopamine levels from being constantly up and down. We should be doing that for ourselves. At the end of the day, all those mini stresses use our system's ability to be able to recover safely.

'INFLAMM-AGEING' AND THE LINK BETWEEN INFLAMMATION AND STRESS

We've briefly touched on inflammation already and we'll be going into more detail on page 134, particularly with the role inflammation plays in gut health. Primarily, inflammation is a healthy response to injury or illness. 'Inflammation is the immune system doing what it needs to fight off what it thinks is a foreign invasion: whether that's bacteria, viruses, surgery or an injury,' says Dr Ravindran (i.e if we cut ourselves and the skin becomes inflamed or red). But we're increasingly hearing about how too much inflammation in the body can lead to a host of wider health problems. 'Our present research is very much revolving around the concept of inflammation being at the root of many long-term conditions,' says Dr Deepak Ravindran. 'Even the medical community is taking time to get its head wrapped around, because we always think of inflammation as a process and something that is done at that time by the body to protect itself.'

One of these things is something called: 'inflamm-ageing'. 'The skin is a dynamic and important organ in itself with its own immune system,' says Dr Ravindran. 'Acute inflammation can occur with external forces, e.g. an acute sunburn, but also a chronic low-grade inflammation that can have a significant adverse impact on the skin. Inflamm-ageing is now being recognized as a key player in other age-related conditions but can be particularly visible when it happens in the skin.'

There can be two factors at play when it comes to premature ageing. 'Photo-ageing' is caused by external ultraviolet (UV) rays and repeated exposure can activate an inflammation response in the skin, causing things like pigmentation, sun spots and coarse wrinkles.

DR RAVINDRAN'S
STRESS-BUSTING TIPS

1. OPTIMIZE YOUR SLEEP

'Good sleep will actually help your immune system wash out any inflammatory chemicals in the brain,' says Dr Ravindran.

2. PHYSICAL ACTIVITY

Movement helps to change the nerve circuits in our brains and has a beneficial effect on the nervous system.

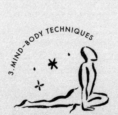

3. MIND-BODY TECHNIQUES

Meditation, gratitude practices, cold water exposure (if you have no underlying health conditions) and yoga nidra [see page 90] can all help to cycle the nervous system back to a place of calm.

The second one is intrinsic ageing, which is caused by internal inflammation. 'This is often accompanied by thinning of the superficial lining of the skin and fine lines of wrinkles, which is due to cell loss and flattening of the layers between the skin,' says Dr Ravindran. 'It can also cause skin conditions like eczema or psoriasis.' The skin can often look dull or unhealthy in the presence of chronic stress. 'Our skin is a reflection of other factors going in the body, due to the impact of environment, sleep and diet,' Dr Ravindran says.

GUT HEALTH AND STRESS

We've made huge strides in terms of our knowledge of wellness and gut health is one of the emerging areas that we now know has a huge impact on our overall wellbeing. It's only in the last five to ten years that scientists have really started to understand the gut–brain connection and have put the time, money and effort into finding out more about it. I think it's important to land that point because often people say to me, 'We hadn't heard of gut health or any issues with it five years ago.' But the truth is that we just didn't know about it! There's so much fresh, amazing knowledge coming out about our gut health, and we owe it to our wellbeing to put a megaphone behind it.

A gut health pioneer that I've been lucky to work with is nutritional therapist Eve Kalinik, author of *Happy Gut, Happy Mind*. 'The gut is both fascinating and compelling in terms of its impact on our overall health and wellbeing,' she says. 'The gut microbiome collectively refers to all the microbes that live in our gut and their genetic material and it is now being considered an organ in its own right, due to its myriad and far-reaching influence over many different systems in the body.' This includes digestion and absorption of nutrients from our food, but it can also have a marked impact on the functioning of our immune system, mood, managing inflammation and hormones. 'Suffice to say what happens in the gut doesn't just stay in the gut,' Eve says.

As well as managing inflammation in the body, up to 95 per cent of serotonin production, aka the 'happy hormone', happens in our gut, along with around 50 per cent of dopamine (another feel-good neurotransmitter) and GABA, which helps to calm our nervous system. The gut also plays a key role in keeping our circadian rhythms and the sleep–wake cycle in check, and even plays an important part in hormonal health. 'There is a subset of microbes in the microbiome called the estrobolome that impacts on oestrogen metabolism,' says Eve. 'Recent research has linked this to changes during the menopause and how one affects the other.'

Laid out like that, we can start to see what a massive influence our gut plays – in all aspects of our health. And one of the biggest influences on our gut health is stress. The gut–brain axis is the signalling system between our gastrointestinal tract and three of the main bodily systems: our central nervous system, our immune system and something called the HPA axis, which stands for the hypothalamus pituitary adrenal axis. The HPA axis also links our hormonal system with the central nervous system and is pivotal in the stress response. In acutely stressful situations, our bodies react by producing a surge in our stress hormones, primarily cortisol and adrenaline, and directing blood away from the digestive system and towards our muscles instead.

This becomes a problem for our gut when that threat response becomes sustained and chronic. Again, this can be a direct result of modern stress and because our primitive sensing systems haven't evolved to differentiate between physical danger and mental stress. This means our stress hormones are being constantly activated and prioritizing the 'fight and flight' response over our body's 'rest and digest' mode, which is essential for good gut health.

WHY IS IT CALLED THE SECOND BRAIN?

Most of us have experienced butterflies in our stomach when we're nervous or anxious and we're all familiar with the term 'gut feeling'. This isn't just a saying: our gut contains extremely sensitive nerves and impulses, which directly influence our mood. Our brain and body are linked by something called the vagus nerve, which is also referred to as the 'information superhighway'. The longest nerve in our body, the vagus nerve runs from the brainstem, through the face and neck, heart and lungs and down into the abdomen. Directly connected to the autonomic nervous system, the vagus nerve is responsible for whether we go into sympathetic (fight or flight) or parasympathetic (rest and digest) response.

A large part of this is down to something called vagal tone, which helps to control functions like our heartbeat and rate of breathing. Healthy vagal tone means better emotional regulation, higher levels of resilience and connection and better physical health. Low vagal tone has been linked to poor emotional regulation and attention levels in children, as well as higher levels of anxiety. The healthier our vagal tone, the more we're able to respond better to stress without going automatically into the fight or flight mode. So how do we strengthen our vagal tone? As the vagus nerve is connected to our vocal chords, things like breathwork (see page 94), singing, humming and even gargling with water have been proven to help.

A BEGINNER'S GUIDE TO THE MICROBIOME

'The microbiome essentially refers to all of the microbes that live on and inside us: bacteria, fungus and parasites,' says Eve. The largest collection of these microbes is found in our gut. 'It's a whole different ecosystem,' Eve says. 'There are literally trillions of microbes in our gut. And most of them are really good for us, so we do want bugs in our gut because they are crucial to our survival.'

The idea of parasites might be a bit grim but healthy ones help us with a range of things, from digesting fat to reducing stress and sugar levels. When we're activating our stress hormones on a regular basis this can change the composition of the gut, which means we get less of the good bugs and more of the bad ones, which in turn can lead to digestive problems and gut-related conditions like IBS.

Poor microbiome health has also been linked to the rise in autoimmune diseases, which, as we talked about earlier in the chapter, predominantly affects women. 'Clinical data and research indicate that there may be an association between gut health and autoimmune conditions such as Hashimoto's disease, psoriasis and rheumatoid arthritis, which is not all that surprising since most of our immune system is located and managed in our gut,' says Eve. 'More recent research has also indicated that people with major depressive disorders may often lack certain microbes in their gut and/or harbour ones that might be pathogenic in nature. There can therefore be an association between the health of the gut microbiome and a possible link to some of these conditions.'

For such a central part of our body, the microbiome is surprisingly fragile. The barrier of our gut is semi-permeable and only one cell layer thick, or approximately 1mm. This is so it can efficiently extract the nutrients we need from our food, but the same sensitivity also makes our gut quite vulnerable. When a gut lining is weakened due to stress or diet, for example, it's more at risk of 'bad' bacteria infiltrating, which can lead to conditions like leaky gut. 'We don't want things that should stay in the gut moving out of the gut, which can include certain pathogenetic bacteria and other pro-inflammatory molecules,' says Eve. This can lead to a systemic inflammation, which puts our immune system on high alert and plays into what Eve calls a 'vicious stress loop' of a compromised gut and systemic inflammation. 'It can essentially feed back into that stress loop, and almost perpetually drive the "fight or flight" response.'

EVE'S GUT-FRIENDLY GUIDE

The *Happy Gut, Happy Mind* author gives us the lowdown on how to supercharge our gut and stay on top of stress.

FOLLOW THE FIBRE

It's no surprise that having a good, balanced diet is key. 'The first thing you need to do is make sure you're having sufficient amounts and diverse sources of fibre in your diet,' says Eve. 'This could come in the form of any plant-based foods: vegetables, fruits, whole grains, nuts and seeds.' The rule of thumb when it comes to fruit and veg is the brighter the better, as they're packed full of health-boosting plant compounds called polyphenols. And you'll want to aim for a mixture of colours. Think 'eat the rainbow'; it sounds a bit clichéd but it is a good analogy.

THE 30-A-WEEK HACK

It's not just about quantity, but diversity. Forget your five a day;
recent research from the American Gut Project shows that getting in thirty different types of plants a week is what we should
be aiming for. If thirty feels like an insurmountable amount, don't
worry. It doesn't mean you have to sit down with the equivalent
of your local supermarket's fruit and vegetable section on your
plate at every mealtime. Nuts and seeds count and a great way to
get a multiple plant hit is a nut and seed mix. 'You can add up
to ten different types in one go,' says Eve. 'Have them easily on
hand to sprinkle over porridge, salads or soups. That's an easy
way to get a diverse amount of plants.'

ROTATE YOUR GRAINS

Adding diversity doesn't have to mean loads of effort and complicated new recipes. Instead, add a twist to what you do already.
'With things like porridge or overnight oats, have three or four
different grains on rotation like oats, quinoa, buckwheat and rye
flakes for example,' Eve says. 'It's still the same formula but you're
just rotating the things in your store cupboard.'

> **Top tip:** Have three different nut butters on rotation
> and add a spoonful to your breakfast every morning.

EAT A FERMENTED FOOD DAILY

Little and often is better rather than having one big portion per
week. If things like kimchi and sauerkraut sound a bit too strong

for your palate on a regular basis, things like unsweetened live Greek yogurt, natural yogurt and some cheeses have good amounts of the probiotics we need for a healthy gut. Hard, aged cheeses contain the most probiotics, so look for things like good-quality Cheddar, Manchego, Parmesan and Gruyère.

PROBIOTICS VS PREBIOTICS

Live cultures or plant fibres? While we're on the subject, it can still feel like there's a bit of confusion around probiotics and prebiotics and what does what, so here is the low down.

Probiotics are essentially live beneficial bacteria and yeast that we ingest through food and supplements. 'Technically probiotics really refer to supplements, but in a food-based form these would be fermented foods, so things like sauerkraut, kimchi, traditional hard cheese, live natural yogurt, kefir and miso,' says Eve. 'I'm generally more of a fan of taking in these through fermented foods as they come wrapped up with other nutritional benefits. However, probiotic supplements can be useful, especially after a course of antibiotics. They won't ever be a panacea for gut health though in my opinion.'

While probiotics feed our microbiome, **prebiotics** act more like a fertilizer. 'Prebiotics refer to a specialized group of fibrous compounds that we find in certain plant foods, or we can also supplement,' Eve says. 'Unlike probiotics, or fermented foods, which we ingest and may cultivate in the gut, prebiotics have a feeding effect on the existing good bacteria in our gut.' We can find prebiotics in foods like garlic, onions, leeks, asparagus, bananas, oats and cashew nuts as a few examples.

In a gut shell:
Probiotics = feed the gut
Prebiotics = fertilize the gut

OMEGA 3

'Omega 3s are a key component in how our body manages inflammation as well as supporting brain health,' says Eve. (Read more on mood-boosting foods in Chapter 3.) Crucially, omega 3s are essential fatty acids we don't make ourselves and have to take through our diet instead. Omega 3 is found in the highest quantities in oily fish, so things like salmon, mackerel, sardines and anchovies.

Organic grass-fed meat is also a source of omega 3. 'Plant-based sources of omega 3 are a different type and are harder for our bodies to convert into the more active form we can utilize, so we do need to compensate for that,' says Eve. 'If you're vegetarian or vegan, top up your levels of plant-based omega 3 with flaxseeds, chia seeds, walnuts and algae.'

SPICE UP YOUR LIFE

Another easy way to manage inflammation and increase diversity is to get in lots of spices. 'When we talk about plants, it's not just talking about fruits and vegetables,' says Eve. 'Spices and herbs, both fresh and dried, are often very high in their polyphenol and anti-inflammatory benefits.' Dried herbs and spices are also much more concentrated than fresh herbs: the general rule of thumb is a teaspoon of dried herbs to a tablespoon of fresh herbs.

Lots of herbs and spices are powerful antioxidants, which means they help to neutralize free radicals. These are unstable atoms in our body that can cause oxidative damage to our cells, which can cause inflammation, illness and premature ageing.

Try these anti-inflammatory herbs and spices:

* Ginger
* Garlic
* Turmeric
* Cardamom
* Black pepper
* Rosemary
* Cinnamon

THE LINK BETWEEN SUGAR AND STRESS

We all love a bit of sugar and I'm never one to turn down a good slice of birthday cake, but the research shows that there is a link between sugar and stress. Lots of us reach for something sweet when we're up against it or need a bit of comfort, which can play into a different type of stress loop. 'When we eat sugar, it triggers a dopamine hit in our brain, which is our reward hormone,' says Deirdre Egan, a registered nutritional therapist and women's health coach specializing in midlife health and stress. 'It makes us feel happy, which makes us more likely to repeat the behaviour again.'

Stress can increase our blood glucose levels. As our primary stress hormone, cortisol's main job is to regulate our body's response to stress. Being in a constant stress state means our bodies are producing more glucose to keep up with the energy output, which increases our appetite. 'This makes us crave even more sugar than we originally needed to get that dopamine hit,' says Deirdre. 'That little bit of sugar isn't going to do the trick any more. We want more and more.'

So how can we avoid becoming a permanent passenger on the sugar-stress rollercoaster? Being aware of our emotional triggers is a good starting place, says Deirdre. 'What is it that makes you reach for the chocolate or biscuits? Is it tiredness? Is it that you go into a stress response when your boss gets angry? It's about bringing awareness to it and thinking: "Okay, how can I manage this differently?"'

It's not about completely banning sugar from our diet though (hallelujah). Some studies suggest that willpower is a finite source and if constantly drawn on, we're more likely to run out of it. Other research has shown that willpower is more about building long-term habits than having iron control. And that includes choosing when to say yes and no to sugar. 'Even speaking as a nutritionist, I don't believe in not having any sugar,' says Deirdre. 'If somebody's made a homemade cake, that's a mindful, "good for the soul" thing and a shared experience with friends. The difference with sugar cravings and emotional eating is that generally we don't feel very good afterwards and it has a psychologically bad impact.'

Deirdre's healthy ways to hit the sweet spot:

1.   If you really need something sweet, try and eat it after a meal because that has less impact on your blood sugar and you're going to get less of a rollercoaster.

2.   If you are craving something sweet, try this simple go-to. Take a Medjool date, remove the stone and have it with a blob of almond butter and a square of really dark chocolate. Not only does it taste good but you're also

getting fibre in the date, healthy fats in the almond butter and antioxidants in the dark chocolate. It will spike your blood sugar a little bit but not as much if you have it with a meal, and secondly, you're still getting some goodness and not just that empty calories effect.

WHY NATURE IS THE PERFECT ANTIDOTE TO STRESS

Humans and the natural world are part of the same ecosystem; yet, as we discussed in the Sleep chapter, modern life has seen us lose that innate connection. Seasons can roll by without us even really noticing. With the pace of life as it is these days, we can feel like we haven't got the time, or even the inclination, to seek out some green space.

The thing is, humans have a primal craving to be in some sort of nature. And the longer we go without it, the more we feel the effects of deprivation. The wellbeing world is constantly brimming with new ideas and innovations, but the flipside is that we can overlook what's in front of us – and that's the powerfully restorative effects of being in nature.

I do consider myself an outdoorsy person but some days I still have to consciously make it a priority to get outside, even if it's for 10 minutes. No matter how grim the weather is, or how much I've got on, I know 100 per cent of the time that getting out for some fresh air will make me feel at least 10 per cent better. I work in London two days a week and if I'm having one of those days, or things can feel like they're piling up a bit, I go for a walk along the river Thames. The size of the river and looking across the horizon to take in the skyline is a great way of putting any of my problems into perspective. It might sound like such a small thing, but it's a brilliant head clearer for me. It always pays off, whether it's a bit more energy in the afternoons or pressing the brake on a busy day and having time to pause, decompress and think.

The natural world is of huge importance to us at NEOM. From using the purest high grade essential oils in our products, to incorporating nature in our wellbeing practices, to becoming a certified B Corp business and putting the planet first, sustainability is at the heart of everything that we do. I really am so passionate about both driving and strengthening that symbiotic link between us and the environment. It's a reciprocal relationship. The modern world with the invention of emails and Zoom calls might have damaged our connection in many ways, but a bit of feel-good greenery is always available if we look hard enough, and we can instantly reap the benefits.

The power of nature on our wellbeing is backed by science, too. There are literally thousands of studies about the restorative effects on humans, from reducing anxiety and depression to better concentration levels and stronger immune systems. Ecopsychology is a growing therapeutic field based on the psychological benefits of nature, while forest bathing or *shinrin yoku*, the ancient Japanese art of immersion in nature, has gone mainstream in the UK and is even being prescribed by some doctors and GPs to boost patient wellbeing.

A University of Sussex study found that the sounds of nature can physically alter our brain connections, reducing our fight or flight instinct and increasing the parasympathetic rest and digest response instead. Participants listened to both natural sounds and artificial environments (e.g. a busy street with traffic noise) and had their brain activity and heart rates monitored. It was found that listening to nature was associated with more outward-focused attention, i.e. engaging more with the physical environment, while listening to sounds of artificial environments promoted more inward-focused attention associated with overthinking, anxiety and worry.

A 2021 US review from the Proceedings of the National Academy of Sciences (PNAS) looked at eighteen studies investigating the health benefits of natural sound. They found that water sounds, such as a gurgling brook or a waterfall, tended to be the most effective at improved positivity, while bird sounds were best for lowering stress. It doesn't even have to be the real thing: participants listened to recordings of nature sounds in laboratory settings. So even if you can't get out into nature, listening to nature sound apps or soundtracks is still a proven way of lowering stress levels.

When it comes to stress in particular, research shows that nature is one of the most effective antidotes there is. Studies measuring the levels of cortisol in people's saliva before and after time spent in nature reported lower levels of stress hormones and lower blood pressure, as well as better immune system function, reduced anxiety and even higher levels of self-esteem. A study of 20,000 people by Exeter University found that 120 minutes was the amount of time people needed to spend in green spaces per week for improved health and wellbeing. It didn't matter whether participants broke up the time into chunks or did it all at once, but 2 hours was the minimum time (people who didn't meet that threshold spending time in nature reported no obvious benefits).

Ask me anything

Q: I see a lot about CBD (cannabidiol) and how it's meant to help anxiety. Have you tried it and what did you think?
A: CBD hasn't worked for me personally (but I know people for whom it has). I think the problem is that the research into its

effectiveness is still in fairly early stages compared to other products and it's quite an unregulated area, so the products can differ wildly. If you are interested in trying it, my advice would be to choose products that have clear evidence-based claims behind them.

A WINDOW OF WELLBEING

A joint UK and New Zealand study found that having a window with a view of greenery improved cognitive function and concentration levels and reduced stress at work. Researchers proposed that the presence of a window allowed for 'micro-restorative experiences' and that 'indirect nature experiences provide a broad range of health and wellbeing benefits'. So even if you can't get outside physically, having a green view can help reduce stress and improve focus, which in turn has a bonus de-stressing effect.

MY NATURE BOOK PICKS

As I've mentioned previously, I'm a big bookworm and one of my favourite topics is our connection with the environment and the natural world. There are some really gorgeous nature books out there and these are some of my favourites in my bookcase and in the kitchen:

1. *The Wild Journal: A Year of Nurturing Yourself Through Nature* by Willow Crossley

2. *Wintering: The Power of Rest and Retreat in Difficult Times* by Katherine May

3. *How to Eat Brilliantly Every Day* by Abel & Cole

4. *Every Day Nature* by Andy Beer

5. *Rewild Your Mind* by Nick Goldsmith

ANXIETY

Stress and anxiety often go hand in hand and when you're in the thick of it, it can be hard to differentiate between the two. Anxiety can come in many guises: health anxiety, climate anxiety, social anxiety, anxiety about public speaking, anxiety about driving, even anxiety about getting anxiety, which is something I can definitely relate to. One thing that's always helped me is having a plan B or plan C in case the intended plan A doesn't go right, or something gets in the way. For example, if I'm going to an event or party and I'm feeling tired, instead of getting anxious about it myself, I will just tell myself I can leave at any point I choose to. Just having options or that get out of jail card makes me feel better. Whatever the situation, once you've got comfortable with your plan B, C (or even D), you might even feel good sticking with plan A after all, because you know you've got options.

Someone who's really helped me with my own anxiety is author of *Untangle Your Anxiety* and registered psychotherapist Joshua Fletcher, who specializes in the field of anxiety disorders and stress management. Josh suffered with his own crippling anxiety and panic attacks, and he's just got a really good breadth of advice, whether you are a serious anxiety sufferer or you just get a bit panicky before you go into a meeting.

JOSHUA FLETCHER'S 'ANXIETY 101'

There are two types of anxiety and I'm very passionate about separating the two. The first type is your **conventional outward anxiety**. It's a type of anxiety that everyone can relate to: 'Oh, I'm nervous about my job interview. I'm nervous about my first day, I'm nervous about my son starting school, I'm nervous about a medical appointment, or getting a tooth removed.' That's the anxiety that isn't tarnished by any taboo. It can feel a bit debilitating, but it's the kind of anxiety that you can share with everyone, and everyone gets it, no matter where you're from, or how old you are. You could have legitimate worries in your life like financial worries or health worries, or you might be grieving, or maybe you're going through a horrible divorce. Anxiety will be there, but it's the product of a stressor.

The second type is **inward disordered anxiety**. This is the anxiety that often goes unspoken. It's very inward and excessive and can involve catastrophic thoughts that feel real and intrusive, or thoughts that are taboo in nature and usually conflict with your morals. This kind of anxiety is characterized by things like panic attacks, excessive compulsions and reassurance seeking. It's where the majority of your day is dictated by a sense of unease and doom, and you don't feel like your usual self. Conventional anxiety is arguably part of your normal self. But when anxiety becomes excessive and disordered and consumes you, then that's when it becomes a problem. It's a bit redundant when people say, 'I have anxiety.' As a therapist, I would always want to know, what kind of anxiety? There's a pick 'n' mix of how it presents.

HOW TO CHARACTERIZE ANXIETY

I break anxiety down into three columns. In the first column you've got **thoughts**. You notice an anxious thought start to appear: *What if . . .?* Everyone can relate to those. Then you get the very common but more serious ones: *I should . . .* If you're someone who has interminable to-do lists, who feels guilty for resting, never finishes that to-do list, always adding and beating themselves up for not feeling productive, feeling guilty for prioritizing yourself . . . that is a form of anxiety and it's something that can be addressed. And then comes: *I can't . . .* People avoid things and don't go for them because they're afraid. Total avoidance is usually due to self-esteem, fear of rejection, fear of abandonment, fear of fear itself, so these are the thought patterns that reoccur: what if/I should/I can't.

In the second column you've got **feelings**. Feelings of unease, terror, doom, irritation, a horrible sense of foreboding. It can be anger, sometimes it can be grief or sadness, or it can be just feeling nervous or on edge. All of that is on the anxious spectrum. If someone says: 'I've had anxiety,' I'd ask, 'What does it look like?'

Lastly there are **sensations**, the physical and psychological. It could be a tight chest, or you can't quite catch your breath, or you've got a lump in your throat. Your heart might be pounding, you may be sweating, feeling light-headed, or you feel detached or disassociated. I get my clients to describe what their anxiety looks and feels like. This might sound something like this: 'Allright, well, actually recently I've had a lot of "what ifs" and I'm not having panic attacks as such, but it's a sense of unease that follows me around. And I've noticed that in my chest and in my posture.' If we can characterize our anxiety, we start to look at it subjectively and understand what's happening, rather than letting it overwhelm us and seeing everything through the lens of anxiety.

ANXIETY ISN'T DOWN TO UNCERTAINTY

It's what your brain perceives as a threat, because everything is uncertain. Anxious people are happy doing uncertain things. Anxious people go to work. It's not uncertainty people are afraid of, it's threat and that can differ from person to person. For example, I like socializing, so my brain does not perceive people as a threat. Whereas someone who has been bullied or neglected by their parents might see people differently. Their brain has remembered the threat, so socializing is going to feel a threat for them. (See pages 57, 136 and 138 for more about stress and the fight or flight response.)

EXCESSIVE ANXIETY IS DOWN TO
AN EXHAUSTED NERVOUS SYSTEM

A lot of anxiety thrives off stress. If you're really stressed but you never prioritize yourself, you're just going stay in the stress anxiety cycle. Mine certainly started that way. I was just really stressed and I didn't stop. Then one day I had a massive panic attack at work. In hindsight, I was like, 'Oh yeah, that was really coming, wasn't it?' But I didn't know what was going on. That's the scary bit of anxiety, so learning about what's happening in the body is really important, and makes it less scary. It's absolutely okay to say to yourself: 'Right, I'm going to prioritize me now.'

ANXIETY INVOLVES CORTISOL

Know that when you're feeling tense, that's just adrenaline; when your heart is pounding, that's adrenaline. If your mind's racing, that's your threat response and the effects of adrenaline and cortisol. I often talk about morning anxiety and waking up with a feeling of dread. That's just too much cortisol release. Anxious people who are stressed and with very sensitized nervous systems have more cortisol in their systems in the mornings. You wake up, your body 'pings' and your head fills with doom and gloom. When you explore your thoughts through the lens of cortisol, everything's horrible, so I sit there and tell myself: 'That's just cortisol.' I find that knowing stuff like that is really helpful in knowing my brain state. If you're worried about what people think of you, remember that this is just a threat response system. That it's not you, it's your anxiety. What would your non-anxious version think?

IF YOU'RE EXPERIENCING ANXIETY
MY ADVICE WOULD BE . . .

I'd always recommend therapy. Having a safe space to talk with someone neutral can be really helpful. Obviously do your due diligence and contact your GP as a first port of call, but do explore other options if you don't feel you are being heard. Find the right information. Be around people who are unconditional, if you can find them. Remember your boundaries; if you find yourself in a stressful environment, know that it's okay to prioritize yourself.

IF SOMEONE ELSE IS EXPERIENCING ANXIETY MY ADVICE WOULD BE . . .

Anxiety is literally fear. So if someone is choosing to still do things that the non-anxious version of them would do, that's the definition of courage and bravery. Also, remember that anxiety isn't a switch. Once adrenaline and cortisol have been released, no amount of telling someone to calm down will work. There are no easy fixes but what you can do to help someone is just say, 'It's okay, anxiety always passes. It really will.' Bring them back into the moment. If you're at a party, talk about what you talk about at a party. If you're out in the park, look at what's in the park.

AND FINALLY . . . HOW TO DEAL WITH 'HANGANXIETY'

Hangover anxiety is when your sympathetic nervous system is tired because it's been processing alcohol and your organs have been working a lot. We know the dangers of drinking, but if drinking alcohol is something that you enjoy and can do it in moderation and a safe amount, you don't necessarily need to stop. Hanganxiety is part of social anxiety, where you find yourself ruminating and going over something again and again. Did I say something? Did I offend someone? What did that person's facial expression mean? Were they feigning boredom? If you've spent much of your life placating others, you might want to look into the reasons why. Otherwise trust your instinct and intention. You didn't walk around pouring drinks over people's heads so if you're experiencing those fears – 'What did I say, did I offend?' – it could be a conditioned response.

BREATHING

Breathwork has become massively popular in the past few years because of its proven benefits for reducing stress. One expert I absolutely love in this space is Stuart Sandeman, Breathpod founder and author of *Breathe In, Breathe Out*. Stuart is a super lovely soul and you just feel more relaxed in his presence, whether in person or on one of his Instagram breathwork sessions. According to Stuart, the power of breathwork can be transformational. 'For me, it's the most empowering and powerful tool we have to manage ourselves throughout the day, whether that's for energy, stress, focus or relaxation,' he says.

> **'By taking control of our breathing,
> we can control our stress.'**

Interview with the expert: Stuart Sandeman

Q: How does stress affect our breathing?
A: Breathing and stress are intrinsically linked. Our stress response is triggered by something that is happening around us. The brain sends a signal to our body to create a stress response and part of that stress response is a change in our breathing and heart rate. This can manifest in different ways – short shallow breathing, faster breathing, erratic breathing or unconscious breath holding. If this becomes habitual, our breathing pattern might be the thing that's causing us stress in the long term. It's a bit like muscle memory. So we can have immediate stress happening, or it might be our breathing pattern that's causing us

stress. We can get stuck in a stressful breathing pattern but the good news is that we can also break that stress response through using our breath.

Q: How does it help?
A: Breathing correctly supplies your cells with the energy they need to function. But it's not just about oxygen; you need the correct balance of carbon dioxide to optimize your body's chemistry, so that you can find coherence in heart rhythms and brain function.

Q: Aside from actual stress, what else can affect our breathing?
A: Our clothes – for example, if you're wearing really tight, high-waisted jeans, your diaphragm is not going to be able to descend downward, so you're left to breathe just with your chest. That means that only your chest is moving and the breath pattern is faster than when you use your diaphragm. Simply because of your clothing, you can be stuck in a fast breathing pattern and feeling stressed, even though there's nothing actually stressing you. The wrong size bra can also constrict breathing.

'We can get stuck in a stressful breathing pattern.'

Q: Is there anything else we should be mindful of?
A: Posture is another big one. If you're sitting hunched over at your desk all day then your breathing becomes collapsed. This is also how people can get trapped into dysfunctional breathing patterns. When the breathing is trapped in this stress state, it's constantly sending an alarm bell to the mind. So you could be sitting on the sofa thinking: 'Everything's good but I feel so anxious.'

Q: Breathwork for stress is something we've talked about quite a bit. What technique would you recommend?

A: A phrase I like is, 'If in doubt, breathe out.' The technique I always use is: breathe in for four, hold for four, breathe out for eight. Even doing one cycle you will probably start to notice if you're clenching any muscles or body parts, or if your shoulders are tense. I usually say go for 3–4 minutes if you can. We often have this tug of war going on between our thoughts and us taking control and slowing things down. To break that loop we can either change our thoughts, which is easier said than done because they're so habitual, or we can just override our breathing pattern. Because we have control of our breath, we can take control of our stress in that moment, and the longer and the more we practise it, the better we get at it.

Give it a go:

1. Breathe in for 4 seconds, through the nose.

2. Hold your breath for 4 seconds; keep calm and still.

3. Breathe out for 8 seconds, through your mouth; let everything relax.

4. Repeat.

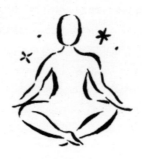

FINAL THOUGHTS

My aim with this chapter was to reframe the idea of stress and to make it easier to understand a) why it happens and b) how it can physiologically show up in our bodies. I think once we get that, the path forwards feels a lot clearer and much less overwhelming. I hope you've got loads of ideas and inspiration now to build your own toolkit, but the one thing I will say again is this: stress prevention is much easier than trying to cure it. It took years of working through my anxiety to understand that. I've now built a lifestyle around keeping my stress in check and it means I can honestly get the best out of life in a million different ways.

The other major thing I've learned through building my own stress toolkit is that self-care is a necessity and not a luxury. It has probably been the greatest gift I've ever given to myself. What I need changes over time, but the basic elements will always be the same: How am I moving? How am I learning and growing? Who am I spending time with? What am I putting into my body? How am I connecting with nature? What am I doing to unwind and take a pause throughout the day? Creating this toolkit has made me feel like I have actual control over my life and how I feel. I'm really excited for you to start building yours and to enjoy reaping the benefits, too.

3.
ENERGY

WHAT IS NATURAL ENERGY?

Natural energy is a term that I use to describe firing on all cylinders. For me it means I am operating at my own personal best. I've got enough physical energy, and my attitude is also the best it can be. I'm enthused about taking on the day, project, challenge – whatever it is. I don't really need to power myself up with coffee or feel the need to prop myself up with chocolate to get me through to the end of the day (although let's be clear, having a bit of chocolate is never a bad thing). It's about hitting my stride and having those pockets of brilliant can-do energy, where everything just comes more easily and feels more joyful. I'm up for it, come what may. There might still be problems, but they feel less of a problem and not insurmountable. It's that ultimate 'seize the day' feeling.

This feeling of natural energy should be easily available to us all, but it's one of the pillars of wellbeing we can sometimes struggle with. We live in a perpetually tired world. Feeling exhausted now is so common that it has its own acronym, TATT, which stands for 'tired all the time', according to the NHS. Three in five Americans say they feel more exhausted than ever, with many citing spending too much time at home and interrupted sleep schedules since the pandemic. A recent YouGov poll found that a quarter of adults felt tired most of the time, 33 per cent felt tired some of the time and 13 per cent of UK adults are permanently exhausted.

Just like with stress, women are also more likely to feel tired than men. In the same survey three in five (61 per cent) say they feel tired when they wake up, even when they get a lot of sleep, compared to around half (49 per cent) of men. Women are also more likely to say they feel like they don't have enough time in the day to rest and relax (49 per cent compared to 44 per cent of men). A 2021 YouGov survey on families and the labour market revealed that employed women with dependent children spent more time on unpaid childcare (an average of 85 minutes per day) and household work (an average of 167 minutes per day) compared to employed men with dependent children (56 and 102 minutes per day) respectively.

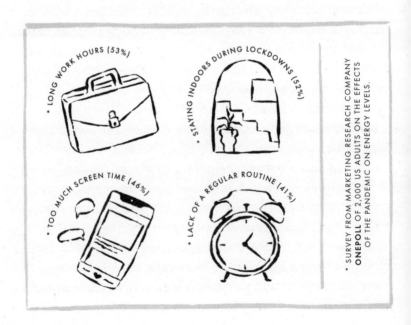

Among the participants working from home in the One Poll survey 34 per cent also said many of the activities that typically boost their energy levels weren't possible during the pandemic, while three out of five respondents said video conferences were more draining than in-person meetings.

> Unlock your energy: What working practices have you inherited from the pandemic? What could you change up to give you more energy?

My energy starts with quality sleep. I can't function at anything nearing an optimum level without it. Once the sleep is in place, it's about feeding myself with the right things and eating a very nutrient-dense diet (factoring in the odd allowance, obviously). This means as much fresh produce as possible, keeping it diverse and focusing on slow-releasing foods that sustain my energy for longer, so complex carbohydrates like sweet potato (my go-to winter dish is a root veggie tray bake), as well as protein on my plate at every meal, so things like salmon, free-range eggs, the odd bit of organic grass-fed meat, topped up with nuts and seeds wherever possible: in salads, stir fries and added to my breakfast smoothie or morning porridge (read more about protein boosting foods on page 100).

As we've already talked about in previous chapters, light is also crucial when it comes to feeling like you're firing on all cylinders and that means getting as much natural daylight as possible. Since starting our brilliant 11 Golden Rules for Better Sleep (see page 45), I've made it a new habit to get outside for a few minutes first thing when the light is at its most potent, no matter the weather or circumstances. Sleep, food and light are my bedrocks and if they're not in place, I know my energy levels will take a dip. Energy can feel like a bit of an intangible thing to grasp, as are the reasons *why* we feel depleted, but like every pillar in this book, there are always some easy and achievable ways to becoming your best energetic self again.

The Energy Edit: My toolkit essentials:

1. A good night's sleep. I can't pour from an empty cup.

2. A 20-minute walk in daylight before 10.30am

3. 1–2 really good freshly roasted coffees before midday.

4. Body brushing in the shower every morning. Great for circulation and getting the blood pumping; I use it with our zingy Super Shower Power Body Cleanser for a double energy boost. I get to work with our Focus The Mind Essential Oil Blend drifting out of my Wellbeing Pod.

5. Exercise or some form of movement always gives me a boost. If I can do it in fresh air, even better.

6. What I call a really hardcore porridge for breakfast. This would be whole oats, chopped banana, honey, peanut butter, raisins and nuts and seeds. It still feels sweet and comforting but gives me lots of slow-release energy.

> *That's interesting*
> Did you know that being dehydrated by just 2 per cent impairs concentration and memory? Those were the findings published in a study by the *Journal of the American College of Nutrition*. Make sure you're getting your 1.5 litres (6–8 glasses) of daily fluids recommended by the NHS – tea and coffee count too!

MIDLIFE OVERCOMMITMENT

The sandwich generation, or 'caught in the middle generation', refers to the age where we find ourselves just as concerned about older parents as we are about our children or teenagers. Suddenly we're the grown-ups and responsible for the various needs of others. It's yet another pressure point and one of the things we've heard many times from customers is that women especially seem to suffer from low energy in midlife. If you are in that position, I think you have to recognize that your importance for your wider family is perhaps now the greatest it's ever been, and that means you have to also start recognizing that your needs are important, and not a luxury. One of the biggest buyers of our wellbeing boxes are older mums who are buying for their daughters who are now mothers themselves. One of the reasons those mothers aged sixty-plus come to NEOM is because they've typically got a daughter who might be in her thirties or forties, who is working super hard, looking after younger children and juggling everything. This isn't by accident either – these are the people who need quick, easy ways to increase their energy when they are being pulled in a million different directions.

So there are plenty of reasons why we can feel like our energy is zapped –aside from a bad night's sleep – and these are true for everyone. However, this was constantly being fed back to us on extreme levels from our customers; once again, we found that women seem to suffer with low energy levels, particularly in midlife. We spoke to hormone specialist Professor Annice Mukherjee to find out why. Dr Mukherjee ran an NHS diagnostic treatment clinic for chronic fatigue for over a decade and has seen what she calls a 'paradigm shift' in the number of midlife women suffering with lack of energy and exhaustion.

Here are the key learnings from a recent conversation I had with Annice, on why trying to manage the 'uber juggle' of midlife can leave us feeling wiped out.

1. **Out of the thousands of patients I've seen over the years, it has been predominantly women presenting with chronic fatigue**. Complex medical fatigue is more often seen in women's health and chronic fatigue is three times more common in women than men. Autoimmune disease is twice as common in women than men and is where the body starts to fight against itself. Oestrogen has a complex effect on the immune system. Many autoimmune disorders tend to affect women during periods of extensive stress on the body such as after pregnancy and during menopause. Chronic stress has a detrimental and suppressive effect on your immune system and your wellbeing. One of the biggest issues I see in women suffering from chronic fatigue is over-commitment. This is particularly common in midlife at a time when hormone changes (perimenopause) are also happening. It's unrelenting standards, it's wanting to be

everything to everybody and do everything for everyone, it's very low self-care. You just take on more and more.

2.   **One term I always use in my chronic fatigue service is boom or bust**. Your body *can* make energy and push you through by producing extra cortisol and stress hormones. It *can* get you through challenging times even when you haven't got energy in your tank, but at some point, your body will say no. It's like an energy overdraft: you constantly go and try and take more out than you have, and you can do it for a while, but then it's a bit of a 'computer says no' scenario and you crash and can't do anything afterwards. This is a really common scenario I see with overcommitment, especially in women. It's such a false economy.

3.   **Over the last ten years there has been a complete paradigm shift.** Burnout and fatigue are much more prevalent now and it's become almost normal. Around 15 per cent of consultations in primary care are coded as 'tired all the time'. We go to the doctor thinking there's got to be something seriously wrong because we're permanently exhausted. And it's true, there is something wrong, but it might not be what you think. It might not show up on routine tests!

4.   **The easy bit is the diagnostics.** People present with exhaustion, fatigue, weight gain and other non-specific problems, or think they've got a thyroid problem because they have also gained weight. We can run all the tests and do a scan but time after time, they come back normal. It's not because there's nothing wrong but because the

homeostasis, which is our body balance, has gone out of sync. This isn't to dismiss these symptoms but rather show that the solution isn't in medical action and that subtle changes to our lifestyle can add up and have a big impact.

5.   **Loss of energy is not straightforward.** There are many factors involved; it can be hormones, gut health, physical activity level and conditioning, adrenal stress imbalance, perimenopause and lifestyle factors like over-exposure to blue light at night and consuming stressful content 24/7. But one of the overriding factors is overcommittment. People are pushing their body so that it can't cope, and their stress response becomes dysregulated. This all links to the cortisol response: when your cortisol is too high, your immune system doesn't work as well. You're more susceptible to minor bugs and other things, and when you're unwell you feel more fatigued. Hormones do play a role, but it's almost never just one system.

6.   **When I talk to patients it never ceases to amaze me how much is going on in their lives.** The menopause comes at a time when women have often been overcommitted for years. Menopause can be the issue but often everything gets blamed on it, when actually, it's a lot to do with other things. It's looking at lifestyle factors and eating a nutritious diet filled with whole foods, cutting down on excess alcohol, having less screen time and taking regular breaks for movement. Strength training to keep our joints and muscles strong is also really important at this stage in life, as opposed to being sedentary or – at the other end of the scale – overtraining, which is something else I see in overcommitted women.

7. **People want a quick fix but the key is often a back-to-basics approach**. A huge factor of that is self-care and downtime. If we didn't push ourselves so hard all the time, we'd actually be more productive and get less ill. These things are so obvious but we overlook them. Self-care is not being selfish. If we apply self-care and feel better, we're so much better able to look after those around us.

I'm sure that the concept of overcommitment will resonate with a lot of you as much as it does with me. It's no surprise to me when Professor Annice Mukherjee says women are predominantly the ones presenting chronic fatigue – I think many of us are guilty of overcommitting and it's a troubling sign of our times in which we are all pulled in lots of directions. As I talked about right at the beginning of the book, my NEOM journey started because I had been trying to cram too much stuff into my life, which manifested as anxiety and, later, panic attacks (and that was before kids!).

Although I have learned from that experience and become more disciplined about how I manage my time, there are still times when I look at my diary and silently gasp to myself. When it starts to look too hectic, I get out my invisible machete knife (in fact, I am known to work with my team in this way when they get overwhelmed too). There are always hundreds of things on everyone's to-do lists but the hard work (and the skill) is identifying the few really important things that are going to move the dial. It's having the courage to ditch the commitments that aren't essential at that moment in time. That's not to say it's not important or you won't do it in future, rather you just don't have capacity for it *right now*. Learning to say an unapologetic 'no' to colleagues and friends is a difficult but valuable skill to learn, as is knowing how to prioritize the pockets of time that replenish you – hobbies, coffee with friends, a lie-in, an afternoon doing nothing. They aren't you being 'lazy' but are important pieces of the puzzle that give you energy to fulfil the rest.

> **'Self-care is not being selfish. If we apply self-care and feel better, we're so much better able to look after those around us.'**
> – Professor Annice Mukherjee

Six science-backed things for morning energy:

1. For a natural wake-up call, get outside first thing for a burst of morning light. This is when the shorter alerting blue light waves are at their strongest.

2. Roll your yoga mat out and do 5 minutes of gentle exercises or stretching. Studies show that even the gentlest of movement helps to increase our oxygen capacity and boost blood flow around the body, making us feel more energized and alert.

3. Journalling has been proven to help improve focus, boost creativity and reduce anxiety. Try the 'Morning Pages Challenge', the famous daily writing practice by the author of *The Artist's Way*, Julia Cameron, in which you write an uninterrupted stream of consciousness on three sides of paper.

4. Drink your coffee between 9.30am and 11.30am. This is the sweet spot, scientists say, to make the most of caffeine's energy-boosting effects, as it's the time our natural levels of cortisol are starting to drop.

5.　Put on a power playlist. Combined studies have shown that listening to our favourite music can reduce fatigue and increase the feel-good hormone dopamine, which boosts levels of wakefulness.

6.　Turn the shower to cold for 30 seconds. Extreme cold water expert Wim Hof extols the energy-enhancing effects of cold water exposure and research has found that it improves circulation by boosting blood flow, while cold receptors on the skin send electrical impulses to the brain, which can have an antidepressant effect. One of the biggest studies into the benefits of cold showers followed 3,000 people in the Netherlands who turned their shower to cold for either 30, 60 or 90 seconds at the end of their daily shower. After a month, participants reported a 29 per cent decrease in self-reported sickness, although interestingly the duration of the exposure didn't make much difference. So however long you can stand the cold water, it seems that you'll get the same benefits!

Scan the QR code below to listen to our power playlist.

THE most energizing shower EVER

Wake yourself up with NEOM's Super Shower Power Collection, which is super powered by 100% natural spearmint, rosemary and eucalyptus essential oils.

1.   Use the Super Shower Power Body Cleanser for a charge of hydration and a zingy, refreshing morning kick.

2.   For glowing, invigorated skin, try our Super Shower Power Body Polish with upcycled coffee grounds and almond shells, organic oat milk and an uplifting, refreshing scent.

3.   Give your barnet a boost with NEOM's Super Shower Power Shampoo and Conditioner to deeply cleanse and purify your hair and scalp.

GREEN ENERGY

We've already talked about how getting out into nature has proven benefits for lowering stress and boosting our mood (see pages 144–5) but it can energize us too. Being outside in nature makes people feel more alive, says a series of studies published in the *Journal of Environmental Psychology,* with a sense of increased vitality regardless of what we're doing and with whom. Other studies suggest that the very presence of nature helps to

ward off feelings of exhaustion, with 90 per cent of people reporting increased energy when placed in outdoor activities.

It can also make us mentally sharper. A University of Chicago
study found that children who have green spaces near their school
or home have better cognitive development and self-control,
while adults who live in neighbourhoods with more green space
had higher levels of attention levels and functioning.

Don't have a garden or any green on your doorstep? One
Australian study gave participants a menial task to do, which was
broken up by a 40-second break in which the group were either
shown images of a concrete roof or a roof covered with greenery.
They then asked them to resume doing the menial task. After the
break, concentration levels fell by 8 per cent among the people
who saw the concrete roof but rose by 6 per cent for those who'd
seen the green roof. While research generally concludes that for
maximum wellbeing benefits we need to get out in the real thing,
it just shows that even a small dose of nature, IRL or otherwise,
can boost energy and make us more productive.

THE FOUR TYPES OF ENERGY

I believe that energy isn't just one state and can be made up of
different components. I find it helpful to break it down into four
different states: physical, mental, emotional and spiritual. They
all play into the same energy pot and by categorizing them, I find
it easier to make sure that I'm not overcompensating in one area
at the expense of another.

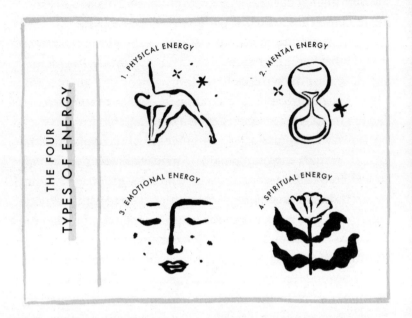

THE FOUR
TYPES OF ENERGY

1. PHYSICAL ENERGY

2. MENTAL ENERGY

3. EMOTIONAL ENERGY

4. SPIRITUAL ENERGY

THE IMPORTANCE OF REST

It might sound obvious to say that to have energy you need to stop and rest, but I think it's worth saying that the key to natural energy is 'purposeful rest', something NEOM's Suzy Reading dives into on page 87. The one thing I've learned over the years is that I function better and achieve better results if I make a concerted effort to stop and refuel the engine with the things that nourish, renew and replenish me. The key difference is that this doesn't just mean passively crashing out on the sofa or hunching over my phone at my desk because I've got nothing left to give. Instead, it means knowing the limits at which I stop being effective, which don't make good use of my time, or anyone else's, and finding the things that actually refresh me.

My high energy day

* I'm a morning person, so I try to schedule the things that require a higher level of concentration and focus earlier on in the day.
* I perform better in short bursts and don't do well in mega long meetings; in fact the NEOM team would say I'm very much a 30 minutes (max) type of woman. We also encourage walking meetings, which are better for problem-solving and creativity.
* Lots of movement. I'll try to get out and about for meetings, to get me out in the fresh air and mix things up in different settings. On a good day I'll fit in a circuits class at my gym, or else it could be taking my Westie Harry Potter to the park, or a lunchtime walk listening to a podcast.
* A good stretch, especially if I've been sitting down for a while. Stretching increases the circulation of blood and oxygen to the muscles and releases tension. For inspiration I like Roger Frampton's book *Stretch: 7 Daily Movements to Set Your Body Free.*
* Learning new things energizes me; in the afternoons I tend towards more reflective things that require less heavy mental lifting, like brainstorming, researching or reading.
* I split my working week between Yorkshire and London Monday to Thursday. Those days can look really busy, but I always have lunch or coffee with a friend on Fridays and finish work at 4pm. Having that gear change is really important and means I don't go into the weekend still in full-on work mode.

Try this
Replacing a sit-down meeting with a stand-up one can reduce the meeting time by 25 per cent, so why not suggest an outside stroll with your coffee in your next catch-up?

ENERGY AND ESSENTIAL OILS

Historically, essential oils have been known for their aromatherapeutic benefits and getting a quick boost of natural energy is one of them. I have different oils in my wellbeing toolkit depending on my energy needs. If I'm feeling lethargic it's more about finding something that will bring me physical energy, so I tend to go for citrussy, bright sparkling fragrances like NEOM's Feel Refreshed scent. But when I need a boost of mental energy for focus, particularly where work is concerned, I'll go for our Focus The Mind, which is a blend of pine, eucalyptus and cedarwood. It's absolutely brilliant and we created it for those intense moments of concentration, for example when you've got to revise for Uni exams or get a work presentation done.

(Want to learn more about how our other natural NEOM products boost our wellbeing? Read the Beginner's Guide to Essential Oils on page 26.)

MOVEMENT

I once walked past a sign for a gym with a quote that read: 'I really regretted that workout. Said no one ever.' I think this sums up the relationship a lot of us have with exercise. We instinctively know that moving our bodies usually makes us feel better, but it can be hard to summon up the energy to get going in the first place. When it comes to physical activity, I think it's about being completely honest about what we will and won't do. Exercise always makes us feel better, but it really shouldn't have to be tortuous or something we actively dread.

When it comes to exercise, I get bored easily, so I commit to two to three times a week at my local circuit class and try and do something else, maybe a home class on the Shreddy App or a longer walk and talk with a friend. I like circuit classes because they tick all the boxes for me: it's a perfect mix of cardio and strength work, which is especially important as we get older. It gets my heart rate up, but not to the point where I'm at my extreme limit, and it always puts me in a positive state of mind afterwards. Crucially, it feels achievable. Because I'm not naturally a sporty person, if I set the bar too high, I won't do it. If someone set me a big target like running a marathon, I would probably do a complete 180-degree turn and end up doing nothing. Whereas if I set the bar lower for myself, I actually end up doing more. Odd but true!

So I think it's really helpful for us to figure out who we are and what our motivation is. For me it's the little bits of movement that I can fold into my day. It's not so much about whether I 'exercise' or not and whether I'm top of the class every time, or smashing a new personal best. It's about having the most active lifestyle I can make for myself, where I feel energized and healthy, without feeling the pressure of having an unrealistic exercise regime to stick to.

JUST GET MOVING

One of the biggest barriers to starting a movement practice can be the belief that we need a dedicated time and place to do it, but physical activity doesn't have to always take place in a gym or a studio. 'It's more about getting your body moving,' says movement and mindset coach Richie Norton (read more on Richie's tips for better sleep on page 71). 'No matter the level of fitness or ability or the age we are, we're trying to cause some sort of physical stimulation and be present in the moment.'

THE NEW HIIT?

We may be familiar with the term HIIT (High Intensity Interval Training) but performing short bouts of VILPA (Vigorous Intermittent Physical Lifestyle Activity) can also boost our health. A study published in *Nature Medicine* looked at 25,000 'non-exercisers' who performed short bursts of activity in everyday life instead, such as doing housework, carrying heavy shopping, walking in quick bursts on the morning commute, climbing stairs or taking the dog to the park. Researchers found that just 3–4 minutes of activity in 'micro patterns' throughout the day had significant health benefits, including better cardiovascular health and longer lifespan.

POWER WALK

Walking is a great way to work on our cardiovascular fitness without being too high impact. 'It gets our heart rate up, works

our joints, lifts our mood and releases tension, which is energizing in itself,' says Richie.

Ten thousand steps a day has become the gold standard
when it comes to our daily step count, but new research shows
that anything between 5,000 and 8,000 steps a day can have the
same health benefits, dependent on our age. When it comes to
walking, Richie says we should be aiming for quality as well as
quantity. 'Think about the pace and intensity. We should be
aiming for feeling slightly out of breath, feeling our heart rate
going up and maybe getting a bit of a sweat on.' As a rule of
thumb, we should use that same metric for any form of exercise
or movement. 'Is it feeling hard? Am I feeling challenged by this?'
says Richie. 'Is my breathing a little bit faster? Am I sweating? If
all of those things aren't happening, we're not working hard
enough and it's too easy.'

MIX IT UP

Changing your workout routine frequently can be beneficial for
both our physical and mental health. A 2015 study published in
the *Journal of Strength and Conditioning Research* found that
participants who changed their workouts every four weeks had
greater improvements in muscular endurance and body composition than those who followed the same workout routine for
eight weeks. If we want a versatile workout that covers all the
bases, what should it look like?

'A yoga workout, strength training exercises with weights
and some cardio is a good mix,' Richie Norton says. 'If we can
find a routine with it where our body feels challenged, that's the
box we need to tick.'

That means regularly updating things. 'We need to change it

as often as we can, so our body doesn't get used to doing the same,' Richie says. 'If we do the same exercise or movement, they no longer challenge those muscle groups and our bodies won't work as hard. Our brain gets used to the same patterns. It knows what's coming, so it can switch off. We get complacent physically and mentally.'

The frequency with which we should change our workout routine depends on several factors, including our fitness goals, our fitness level, our training history and our individual preferences. 'Generally speaking, it's a good idea to change your workout routine every four to eight weeks to avoid hitting a plateau and to continue making progress,' Richie says. 'The frequency with which you should change your workout routine will depend on your individual circumstances, so it's a good idea to consult with a fitness professional to determine the best approach for you.'

FEEL FAB IN FIVE

Haven't got ages to exercise? Don't worry. 'There are studies that suggest that even a short burst of exercise, such as 5 minutes, can provide some benefits,' Richie says. One study published in the journal *PLOS One* in 2014 found that a short burst of high-intensity interval training (HIIT) consisting of just 1 minute of all-out exercise (e.g. cycling or running) followed by 1 minute of rest, repeated five times, improved cardiovascular health and fitness in sedentary men and women. Another study published in the *American Journal of Health Promotion* in 2019 found that just 5 minutes of stair climbing per day improved cardiorespiratory fitness in sedentary office workers.

'These studies suggest that even a short amount of exercise can provide health benefits, particularly if it is done at a high intensity or involves activities that engage large muscle groups, such as climbing stairs,' says Richie. 'However, it's important to note that longer and more frequent bouts of exercise are generally associated with greater health benefits. So while 5 minutes of exercise is better than no exercise at all, it's still important to aim for at least 30 minutes of moderate intensity exercise most days of the week for optimal health.' Again, don't get too particular what it should look like. 'As long as we're doing something that causes our heart rate to lift and we feel physically challenged. And it should be enjoyable.' Want to maximize the wellbeing benefits? 'Do it with somebody else for that social contact and another feel-good win.'

STRENGTH WORK

Not just key for building muscle, strength work also builds bone strength and density. This feeds into an energy loop: the fitter and more capable we feel, the more energy we have to do the things that keep us strong and healthy. This is especially true as we hit the perimenopause and onwards and our oestrogen (which is important for bone health) levels start to drop. If you're not sure how to build up muscle strength, rest assured it doesn't have to resemble an Olympic lifter's workout.

'Strength training can be a variety of things: bodyweight exercises like push-ups, squats or the plank,' says Richie. 'As a guide, it's any exercise that takes you to the point of your maximum effort and strength before your form drops. Take 1–3 minutes of rest before repeating another set of maximum repetitions. Three or four sets is a good target.' Work strength training into your everyday movements: hit the stairs with heavy shopping bags, or hold that kettlebell for that little bit longer.

EASY
ENERGY WINS

*'These are all the different variables we can work with,' says Richie.
'It just has to be something that challenges you in a different way as often as possible.'*

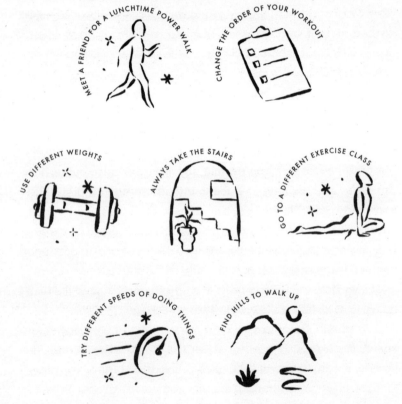

'It's whatever external weight causes your body to shake and that you find hard to hold,' says Richie. Frequency wise: 'Aim for some kind of strength work three to four times a week.'

EATING FOR ENERGY

This is another key place where the 80/20 rule comes in: we all like a bit of comfort food and indulging ourselves every now and again, but it's just making sure that the bulk of our diet is made up of the foods that are going to give us energy to go about our day and help us get the best out of the things we do. Nutritionists say that includes a diet of complex carbohydrates like whole grains, fruit and vegetables, as well as healthy fats from things like fish, nuts, olive oil and avocados. Turn to page 103 to find out the foods that help us feel our best 24/7.

When it comes to a sustainable energy source, protein is at the top of the list. It's important for our long-term energy, as it helps to build and maintain muscles and tissue. It's also what's known as a satiety food as it's denser, which means it takes our bodies longer to digest and keeps us feeling fuller for longer (hence less chance of having an energy dip and reaching for the sugar). Protein is most commonly found in animal products (lean meat, fish, cheese, dairy, eggs) but can also be found in plant-based foods. Top plant protein picks include tofu, tempeh, edamame, lentils, chickpeas, hemp seeds and peanuts. Nutritionist Deirdre Egan gives us some great tips for protein-packed breakfasts on page 187.

Gut health and energy are also explicitly linked. As we discussed in the chapter on Stress, 70–90 per cent of our immune system is located in our gut (see page 137), as well as 95 per cent of our serotonin production, while studies show that an imbalance in the microbiome has been linked to chronic fatigue. You can read more on the microbiome from gut health expert Eve Kalinik on page 134.

DOES FASTING GIVE US MORE ENERGY?

Fasting has become pretty mainstream these days and you probably know someone who does some form of fasting, or maybe you do it yourself. Some of the associated benefits associated with fasting include more energy, better concentration and gut health and stronger immune systems. But is it for everyone?

'There's really mixed evidence on fasting,' says registered nutritional therapist Alice Mackintosh. 'There is a lot of research about the benefits of fasting for things like supporting brain health and its benefits for the gut and inflammation. There's also evidence that some people actually get more stressed when they fast and that it can affect their hormones negatively, so I think there needs to be a dose of caution. Some people really shouldn't be fasting and should check with their doctor before doing it, but other people absolutely love it and it does wonders for their body. I think the main caveat is that everyone is different.'

Most of us fast naturally overnight anyway (hence why the first meal of the day was called 'break-fast'); allowing a 12-hour window overnight gives us all the benefits of fasting and allows our bodies to carry out essential housekeeping duties like muscle and cell repair and cleaning out toxins. 'If you go for four hours between a meal, you could technically say you've been fasting between,' says Alice. 'That's actually a good thing to do. Sticking to breakfast, lunch, dinner, not over snacking, 12 hours of fasting overnight is something we can all benefit from doing.'

WHY DO SOME FOODS MAKE US TIRED?

We know that things like fast food and alcohol can make us feel tired, but why does it happen? 'The impact of what we eat and drink on our energy is just huge,' says registered nutritional and women's health coach Deirdre Egan. 'Fast food is high in sugar, salt and transfats and not what we'd call "proper food". We can be eating all day and still feel hungry, because we're not getting the nutrients that our body needs.'

The lack of fibre and complex natural ingredients in fast food means that our body can break it down and absorb it into the bloodstream very quickly, which causes a spike in blood sugar and then a drop again, leaving us feeling tired and depleted. 'It's also full of preservatives and the "bad" fats which cause inflammation in the body. This impacts our immune system in the long run,' says Deirdre. 'Inflammation is a defence mechanism. Our bodies don't like inflammatory food and it's their way of saying: "I'm not happy and it's not good for me."'

Alcohol might feel like a stimulant but it's actually a depressant. 'We might get a buzz at the time, but alcohol depletes our serotonin and dopamine,' says Deirdre. 'That's when we can get that horrible, anxious feeling, as well as feeling physically bad. Alcohol can also wreck our sleep, so we have the impact of that.'

Ask me anything

Q: What's your best hangover cure?
A: A bacon sandwich and lots of fresh air to focus the mind. I'll also have one of NEOM's energizing Essential Oil Blends pumping out of the Wellbeing Pod, as well as using the Super Shower Power

Body Cleanser, Shampoo and Conditioner. Slathering myself in uplifting zingy fragrances really does help a heavy head to shift.

WATCH OUT FOR SNEAKY SUGARS

We talked about the link between sugar and stress on page 142 and how to avoid the sugar rollercoaster, but sugar can still lurk in surprising places. Granola bars and protein bars are often marketed as healthy snacks, but the truth is often anything but. 'Things like that often have sneaky sugar in them,' says Deirdre Egan. 'It might not say sugar on the ingredients list, but it will have things like fructose, sweeteners or date syrup or rice syrup. All of those things are still going to spike our blood sugar.'

If we want a sustainable energy boost, Deirdre says go as natural as possible. 'It's better to buy a little pack of nuts and seeds, or a protein pot with boiled eggs and spinach if that's more your thing.' Follow this general rule of thumb when it comes to sussing out if a snack is healthy or not: 'You want to be looking out for ingredients that don't make any sense to you and avoiding them.'

Ask me anything

Q: You're known for your love of tray bakes on Instagram. What's your favourite recipe?
A: I don't follow a recipe as such, but my ultimate tray bake is roasting up loads of veggies and popping in some chicken or fish if you want, along with something like cannellini beans. Right at the end I put in a couple of tablespoons of organic cream or crème fraîche for added creaminess, with lots of seasoning – quite often there will be some turmeric in there as well. It can basically be dinner every night on rotation because you can do

different vegetables, different beans, different meats and different herbs and spices.

BREAKFAST ENERGY TWISTS

'An energizing breakfast means a blood sugar balancing breakfast,' says Deirdre. Toast and cereal might be bog-standard but having a brekkie containing zero protein is not going to give us the best start energy wise. 'We want to see colour, complex carbs and healthy fats on our plate but when it comes to sustainability and that slow release of energy, the cornerstone of our breakfast should be protein,' says Deirdre.

Don't want to change your breakfast? Add a few energizing twists instead:

* Add a couple of poached eggs to your wholemeal toast, or a bit of salmon.
* If you have porridge, add some Greek yogurt for protein.
* Add a handful of nuts and seeds to your breakfast cereal – or ideally make your own sugar-free granola. Colourful berries are also a great source of antioxidants.
* If you already start the day on an egg, add a bit of spinach for that extra iron quota.
* Have things like good-quality sausages and bacon in moderation, or half a nutrient-dense avocado.

LET'S TALK ABOUT . . . THE CAFFEINE ISSUE

'To get the most amount of natural energy, we need to find ways to stimulate this other than using artificial means,' says movement expert Richie Norton. 'Our energy can be naturally stimulated but most people have coffee in the morning before they've fired up the endorphins and hormones we can naturally signal to be introduced into our body. This is the caffeine issue.'

This is definitely where the 80/20 mindset plays a part. A moderate caffeine intake has been shown to be supportive of mood, focus and energy, while studies show that consuming two to three cups of coffee a day is linked to a longer lifespan and a lower chance of heart disease. Coffee contains up to 100 biologically active ingredients, including what is called 'cardio protective' benefits that support the heart. (Before you start loading up on the caramel lattes, experts say black coffee with no added sugar is the way to go. Although it doesn't differ too much if it's ground or instant coffee, decaffeinated or normal.)

If you're like me and you love a coffee first thing (sipping it outside, if possible), then great. But if you get up and automatically head for the Nespresso machine, or you find yourself going out for an emergency flat white mid-afternoon to wake you up, doing a bit of gentle movement instead might be better for your energy levels in the long run. 'The more we tap into those practices on a regular basis, the better the pay off,' says Richie Norton. 'They need to be trained like anything else.'

Ask me anything

Q: Is there a natural energy alternative to caffeine?

A: I do like a really good mushroom tea called Lion's Mane by a brand called Dirtea. Studies show that Lion's Mane mushroom contains beneficial plant compounds that help to boost brain health and improve memory and focus, and I definitely find that it helps.

ENERGY AND THE IMMUNE SYSTEM

Dr Jenna Macciochi is a renowned immunologist and author of *Immunity: The Science of Staying Well* and *Your Blueprint for Strong Immunity*. An immunologist is a scientist or medical professional who specializes in the study of the immune system and in particular, Jenna looks at the effects of nutrition and lifestyle on our immune systems. What I really like about her approach is that she demystifies all the science and data and presents it in a relatable, everyday way. 'No matter your starting point, it's never too late to invest in your immune health,' she says.

PROTECT YOUR ENERGY BUDGET

Much like we're advised to manage our finances, we should be taking the same approach with our energy. 'We budget our money over the month and we have to do the same with our energy,' Dr Jenna says. 'If we think about the link between our diet, exercise and lifestyle, the immune systems are really energy intensive.' For example, if we get sick and get a fever, our resting metabolic rate can go up by 10–15 per cent, just trying to fight that fever off. 'This means that our body is consuming much more energy because our immune system is working really hard, which leaves us depleted in other areas,' says Dr Jenna. 'We only have so much energy in the pie. If we're thinking about wellbeing and not wanting to get sick, we can't be burning through our energy budget because there will be nothing left in the pot.' Being 'energy poor' means we don't have the adequate resources to allow our immune system to fight off any bugs or viruses. Meaning we're more likely to be the ones to catch whatever's going about, including any sickness doing the rounds at the start of the school term.

So how can we take care of our energy budget on a daily basis? 'Our energy does come from our diet but the overall equation is looking at the other things draining our energy,' says Dr Jenna. 'It could be mental stress, or it could be that we're just overdoing it with a busy life and not enough rest, alongside trying to go to the gym so many times a week. If we have too much going on one month, we have to pull back and say: "I'm going say no to certain things." It's a "no" to this now so we have the energy to do the other stuff later. Those boundaries are really important.'

DON'T MAJOR IN THE MINORS

Do you have a cupboard full of supplements but no fresh food in the fridge? Are you struggling to remember the last time you went to bed at your ideal time? You could be doing what Dr Jenna calls 'majoring in the minors'. 'We think if we just buy the supplements and energy shakes that's going to fix everything, but that won't make a difference if we're still not sleeping very well and we're rushing around, or if we buy organic food but have no time to prepare it and end up just grabbing food on the go. Certain supplements can definitely help (see page 195) but we have to look at the foundations.'

Ever since Dr Jenna shared her 'don't major in the minors' concept it's stuck with me. It can be so easily done – we buy into the latest influencer ad on Instagram and think we're doing the right thing – so I'm always keeping a check to ensure I've got the foundation of the wellbeing basics like having a good sleep routine, while topping up on the minors, like those in my wellbeing toolkit on page 31.

OUR FEELINGS ARE IMPORTANT

'Nutrition, supplements and extra nutrients are not the only things that support our immune system,' Dr Jenna says. 'It's the body's sensing system, so it's getting inputs from all different things around us, including how we're feeling. We have the empirical data to show that different emotions, such as sadness, optimism and stress, can affect the function of our immune cells. There is a growing body of research that suggests a link between a person's outlook and their immune system. Optimism, which is the tendency to have a positive outlook on life and believe that good things will happen in the future, has been found to be associated with better health outcomes and a stronger immune system.

That's interesting

One study published in the journal *Brain, Behavior, and Immunity* found that people who scored higher on measures of optimism had higher levels of certain immune system markers that help the body to fight off infections and diseases. Another study, published in the *Proceedings of the National Academy of Sciences,* found that people who reported higher levels of optimism had a faster and stronger immune response to a flu vaccine compared to those with lower levels of optimism. 'It's important to note that these studies are observational and don't prove that optimism causes changes in the immune system,' Dr Jenna says. Still, it's pretty fascinating food for thought!

HAPPY MEANS HEALTHIER

'There's some really interesting research on emotions and how well we do in the cold and flu season,' says Dr Jenna. 'Several studies have shown that a person's emotional state can impact their recovery from illness. The connection between emotions and the immune system is complex and not yet fully understood, but research suggests that stress and negative emotions can have a negative impact on the immune system and delay recovery from illness, while positive emotions and a supportive social environment can promote healing.'

I love this concept and it's also super apt at NEOM. When we put an email out a few years ago asking for the best tips for helping wellbeing woes, the favourite answer from the team was 'call a friend' (which is part of my stress busting toolkit, see page 119). During Covid and the whole working from home era, which was pretty intense, I lost count of the times I said this and replaced 'friend' with 'colleague'. It was so important (and something we now just do with our eyes closed) for us to stay connected as a team and lift those up who were feeling really low at the time.

SEASONAL IMMUNITY

Perhaps unsurprisingly, our immune response will vary through-out the year. 'As the seasons change, depending on where we are in the world, the levels of sunlight and temperature change and our bodies compute all this information,' says Dr Jenna. This changes something called our 'gene expression', which if you did GCSE biology you'll know is where the information stored in our genes is turned on to perform a function. 'Throughout evolution we had different germs and more threats to our health during winter than we did during summer,' says Dr Jenna. 'When it starts to get dark in the evenings and the temperature gets colder, our bodies are like, "Okay, we have to prepare for those kinds of challenges."' Adapting with the seasons helps to support our immune systems. 'The produce available in winter like root vegetables often has a lot of the nourishing nutrients that we need to fight off those common winter colds and flus,' says Dr Jenna. It's therefore important to look to nature's bounty to help support our immunity and, in turn, our energy.

That goes for a change of pace as well, and indulging our natural inclination to hibernate during the colder months. 'In the winter we should be battening down the hatches, having cosy evenings with friends and family, relaxing and eating slow-cooked foods,' says Dr Jenna. Instead, it can be the opposite. 'We try and juggle work with Christmas parties and late nights and more alcohol.' On the other hand: 'Summer is a really good time to double down on all those antioxidants and really fresh flavours. There's a lot in moving and eating seasonally, but sadly modern society doesn't recognize that. This disconnect might be why we don't feel our best some or all of the time.'

Dr Jenna's Immune Nourishing Seasonal Soup

* 200g (1 cup) red lentils
* Dash of apple cider vinegar
* Butternut squash (or pumpkin)
* Extra virgin olive oil
* 1 large onion, finely chopped
* 3 garlic cloves, finely chopped
* 1 tablespoon grated fresh turmeric
* 400ml tin coconut milk

* 750ml (3 cups) chicken stock (or vegetable stock)
* 1 teaspoon ground turmeric
* 1 teaspoon ground cumin
* Coriander leaves, to garnish
* High mineral sea salt and black pepper

1. Preheat the oven to 200°C fan.
2. Soak the lentils in cold water with a dash of apple cider vinegar and a pinch of salt, set aside for 10 minutes, then drain and rinse.
3. Roast the whole squash (no need to chop first) in the oven for 1 hour, or until soft.
4. Add a splash of olive oil to a large pan and place over a medium heat. Sauté the onion with some salt and pepper until the onions begin to soften.
5. Reduce the heat and add the garlic and grated fresh turmeric and continue to sauté for a few more minutes.
6. Add the lentils, coconut milk and stock. Bring the soup to the boil, then cover, reduce the heat to low and allow to simmer for 20 minutes until the lentils are soft.
7. Once the butternut squash feels soft, remove from the oven, scoop out the centre (reserving the seeds) and add to the soup.
8. Cook together for a further 10 minutes, then transfer to a blender and whizz until smooth.
9. Meanwhile, rinse the reserved seeds and pat them dry. Add to a bowl with the ground turmeric and cumin and a drizzle of olive oil and toss until coated, then spread out on a baking tray. Roast in the oven for 10 minutes.

10. Serve the soup with a topping of roasted spiced
    seeds, a generous handful of coriander leaves and a
    drizzle of extra virgin olive oil.
(Taken from www.drjennamacciochi.com)

THE CASE FOR SUPPLEMENTS

When I started NEOM back in 2005, people didn't understand the
concept and benefits of using natural-only organic products. It
was perceived by many as a bit like a middle-class badge that
went on a posh carrot and was just something that you paid more
money for. The reality is that a few generations ago, before intensive farming when we ate more locally and seasonally, people
were eating organically just by default. Now it's more typical for
our generation to be eating GM (genetically modified) foods that
are mass-produced to fill the supermarkets for a lower price but
are less nutritious because of the resulting soil depletion of
vitamins and minerals. Organic produce was the norm but a lot
of produce that we see now is a whittled down version of that.
We have to think about these changes to the world of food, compared to where it was seventy years ago, and there's increasing
evidence from multiple studies that many of our fruits, vegetables and grains are a lot less nutritious than they used to be.

Supplements are now part of the wellbeing conversation, but
unfortunately, this area can be a bit like the Wild West. The supplement industry isn't heavily regulated; in many instances, it's
not regulated at all. There's a huge swathe of vitamins and minerals that will just pass through you and make absolutely no
difference. Doing your research and finding a couple of brands
that you really trust is the first thing to do. I only use brands that
are very reputable and have their claims backed up. In terms of

one of the best general websites, Victoria Health is very specific about who they stock and there's a rigorous process, so that's a good place for anyone who's thinking about taking supplements but doesn't know where to start. Brands I like and trust because they are all founded by experts and are transparent about their ingredients and sourcing include Wild Nutrition, Bare Biology, Supernova Living, Equi London, The Naked Pharmacy and Form Nutrition.

Knowing that what you're buying is decent quality and buying from brands who care and source the right things is key. There can be a tendency to start self-prescribing, especially when we're constantly bamboozled with all these amazing health claims in their marketing campaigns. Any reputable brand will have a good customer care service, where they will give you a bespoke prescription and find out what's right for you, rather than just mindlessly selling *at* you. It might cost more but in supplements you get what you pay for and doing it this way can actually end up being more cost-effective in the long term.

The second thing is not taking too much. We can end up with cupboards full of supplements that we never finish or use. Quite often when people start on a supplement journey, they understandably feel like they want to throw the kitchen sink at whatever wellbeing issue they have. The issue with that can be that you start with three, four or five supplements and you're not really sure which ones are working for you and what aren't, or you continue taking all of them forever more, which could cost a fortune. The best approach is to start with one or two and build it up like that. Be mindful of throwing too much at it at the start and keep things simple.

Which brings me on to patience. Timescales can vary from person to person, as well as the level of deficiency we might have in something. For me, it takes about four to six weeks for a new supplement to start to have some effect. 'The caveat is that everyone is different,' says Alice Mackintosh, registered nutritional therapist and co-founder of Equi London. 'Some people might notice changes sooner (especially, say, with their energy levels) but with others it might take longer. The main thing is that you give it three months when taking a new supplement consistently, to really see the full effects.'

So stick with something and don't expect to feel the immediate benefits, otherwise you can spend a lot of time and money hopping around from one thing to another. Also, remember that nothing is a silver bullet. When it comes to supplements, people can fall into the trap of thinking, 'Oh I'm taking that, the problem's gone.' But it has to work in conjunction with everything else.

For example, magnesium plays many crucial roles in the body, such as supporting muscle and nerve function and energy production, as well as helping with sleep, but research shows that large numbers of us don't get enough magnesium from our diet. Lifestyle factors like stress have also been shown to deplete our magnesium levels so, as a result, this is a common supplement that a lot of people start taking in order to improve their energy. But like anything wellbeing-related – and what is certainly the ethos of this book – we have to look at all the factors that could be playing a part in our wellbeing, instead of jumping to a solution.

OMEGA 3 AND FISH OILS

We all need the essential fatty acid omega 3 in our diets, yet we don't always get enough in our diet. I try to eat oily fish, but I don't always eat it as much as I should. For this reason I do take a fish oil supplement and I like a really good-quality brand called Bare Biology. Founder Melanie Lawson experienced postnatal depression after her first child, which was linked to an omega 3 deficiency. Frustrated by a lack of good-quality, sustainable fish oils at the time, Melanie was inspired to start her own brand.

Interview with the expert: Melanie Lawson

Q: Why is omega 3 so important?
A: In a nutshell, omega 3 is needed for all our cells to work properly. A good part of our cell membranes is made of omega 3, particularly in the brain, which is 60 per cent fat. We can't make omega 3, so we have to get it through the food we eat – that's the reason you hear omega 3 referred to as an *essential* fatty acid, meaning that our bodies need it in order to work properly.

Q: Why do we need to take fish oil supplements?
A: Oily fish contains the highest levels of omega 3. In Mediterranean countries people eat things like sardines and anchovies quite regularly, while the Japanese eats tons of oily fish so they are unlikely to need a supplement. But British and American people just don't eat enough oily fish and are deficient in omega 3 for that reason. We might have a bit of salmon here and there but it's not enough. Also, a lot of heavily farmed salmon has increasingly lower levels of omega 3; it's now industry practice to feed salmon with omega 3 supplements to get their omega 3 levels up, which is weird!

Q: What are the key times to supplement with omega 3?
A: A big one is pregnancy and post pregnancy. In order for a baby's brain, eyes and nervous system cells to grow properly the

foetus absorbs something called DHA from mum, which is a type of omega 3. People talk about having 'baby brain', which happens again in menopause when we experience brain fog and can't remember stuff. This can be a sign of omega 3 deficiency, because your brain can't work properly without it. When you breastfeed, your DHA also goes to the baby. That's a critical time when a lot of women become depleted. It can contribute to 'baby brain' at one end of the spectrum right down to severe postnatal depression at the other end. Omega 3 also plays a key role in fertility and there's another type of omega 3 called EPA that is good for that. We have a lot of customers with endometriosis, who've been told by their doctor to take high strength omega 3. It's also anti-inflammatory and can help with arthritis and autoimmune conditions like fibromyalgia.

> '**Baby brain and brain fog are the signs of an omega 3 deficiency.**'
>
> – Melanie Lawson, founder of Bare Biology

Q: How does omega 3 help if we're perimenopausal or have gone through the menopause?
A: It can be the hormonal rollercoaster but it's also quite a tricky stage of life, dealing with teenage kids, getting older, ageing parents. There's a lot going on. Having your brain properly nourished at that point of life is really important, so we don't feel so stressed out or overwhelmed. Omega 3 supports collagen production too, so it's good for skin and hair. Hair loss is something else we can experience in middle age.

Q: What if you're vegetarian or vegan and can't eat fish oil?
A: We do a vegan omega 3, which is made from algae. There is a plant-based source of omega 3 and you can get that from things

like flaxseeds and chia seeds. The problem is that we don't convert it very well to the EPA and DHA version that our bodies need. There are a lot of studies that show that at best, we convert 5 per cent of plant-based omega 3s into the form of omega 3 that we need. So you can find omega 3 in plant-based sources, but fish is the best source.

Q: What should we look for in a good omega 3 supplement?
A: Read the label carefully. For example, a typical high street supplement will say 'High strength Omega 3 1000 mg' (milligrams) on the front. Which sounds great, but if you look at the back and actually read the ingredients and the breakdown, the 1000 mg they're referring to is the weight of the capsules. It might be a 1000mg capsule but may only have a couple of hundred milligrams of omega 3. You need to look at the amount of EPA and DHA – they're the two important ones. Also, look for brands who show transparency. If they don't publish their test results, you have to ask yourself why.

Q: Is there a recognized industry standard for fish oil?
A: IFOS stands for International Fish Oil Standards and it's the only third-party certification programme for fish oils. Every batch is tested for strength, freshness and purity, so looking for things like mercury, arsenic and industrial products and chemicals called PCBs. A lot of people hate fish oil because it repeats on them and gives fishy burps. That's because the oil is rancid. It won't make you ill but it's not great and you don't want to be burping up fish. Most fish oil has a shelf life of two years. Once you've opened them, you'll need to keep them in the fridge and they'll last for a couple of months.

> *That's interesting*
> On a typical day a person uses up 320 calories just to
> think. The brain is the most energy intensive organ in
> the body, contributing to 20 per cent of energy output,
> despite only representing 2 per cent of our overall
> body weight. Studies show that energy consumption
> is mainly in the form of glucose and the bulk of our
> brain's energy budget goes towards sustaining
> alertness and monitoring the environment for
> important information (our neurons firing signals)
> and managing other intrinsic activities such as cell
> health maintenance.

NATURAL SUPPLEMENTS

As we touched on, the supplements industry can be hit and miss
in terms of quality, and this is especially true when it comes to
knowing the difference between natural and synthetic supplement brands. Henrietta Norton is co-founder of Wild Nutrition
and the Food-Grown™ method, which only uses natural nutrients
in their supplements. According to Henrietta, there are some
simple ways to check if supplements have been synthetically
made or if they're natural. An important one is looking at the
names of the ingredients. 'If an ingredient is listed with a chemical
name, it will be a synthetically derived chemical. If you take synthetic Vitamin B1 as an example, its chemical name is thiamine
hydrochloride, which is actually a derivative of the petrochemical
industry and doesn't reflect the format of Vitamin B1 as you would
find it in food. Magnesium stearate is another really common one;

it's a flowing agent that makes the material inside the capsules flow more easily. More naturally derived products will say things like "Vitamin B1 from yeast" or "Vitamin C from citrus pulp".

FINAL THOUGHTS

As I've said before, all four wellbeing pillars are interlinked and energy simply isn't going to be an option for me without a good night's sleep! So, assuming you've mastered that (if not, go back to page 45 and come back here when you have!), you'll always be in a good place to invest in your energy. Of course, our energy levels are hugely dependent on our nutrition and physical activity, but I think it's really valuable to understand that they're also contingent on things like protecting our time and looking after ourselves – remember, the impact of overcommitment is real. We each get our energy from different things, so learn to listen to your mind and your body and add more fun stuff into your life. Say yes more to the right things, but also know when to say a quality 'no' and put your wellbeing first. When we get the balance right, we get more out of those quality moments. Laughter is one of life's great sources of energy and it is the fuel we need to feel like we're firing on all cylinders. When I'm in an energized state, I will honestly get three times more out of my day: I'm way more likely to go to the gym, to get into that flow state at work, to connect with that friend.

Having good energy levels and, in turn, good motivation has probably been the number one driver for me starting my business and pushing it forward every day. I'm not the best at everything but thanks to what I've learned about how to harness my energy, I do always bring enthusiasm to the table and try to spread that around – big time. For me, energy is the secret source of a full and well life. So, remember to feed yours in all the ways you can.

4.
MOOD

Mood has vastly wide interpretations but in this pillar I want to explain how boosting your mood and overall happiness can have an impact on your wellbeing, why it's so important for your overall health, and what you can do to improve it on a day-to-day basis. In many ways this is the trickiest pillar to talk about because, as we touched on in the introduction, happiness means different things to different people.

Again, there is also plenty of interesting evidence that says we have a lot more agency over our happiness than we might think. The numbers vary but research shows that our capacity for happiness is shaped not only by our genetics and external circumstances but also by our intentional activity. Even if we have a predisposition towards certain traits, studies now say those genes may or may not be triggered, and therefore may or may not show up in our lives, depending on what happens to us or how we choose to live. While some people might just be born happier than others, science has given us the hope and the evidence that we have the ability to change our mood state.

The other thing to say about happiness is that it doesn't necessarily mean walking around feeling on top of the world every day. Happiness can be a spectrum of many things: excitement,

We DON'T need to feel 10/10 all the time

pleasure, contentment, satisfaction and joy. We don't need to feel 10 out of 10, all the time. It's more about if you're hovering around a 5/10, how you can make that a 7/10 by reframing a few things and putting some good habits in place. The fact that we have material control over our happiness is incredibly powerful; we just need the tools to know what to do with that control. By arming ourselves with that knowledge and building a toolkit to help us

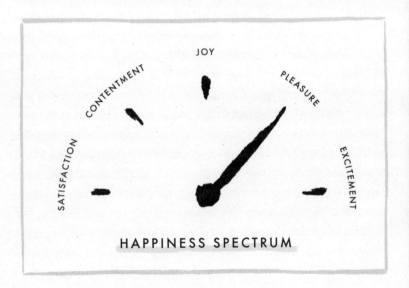

HAPPINESS SPECTRUM

through the ups and downs as they inevitably come along, we will have more agency over our mood and – ultimately – our happiness. We don't need the big things to make us happy. It starts in the here and now, with the small steps.

MY HAPPINESS PHILOSOPHY

WHY THE SMALL THINGS ARE THE BIG THINGS

As I've got older and had more life experience, I've increasingly come to realize that 'the small things are the big things'. By which I mean the things that are within our control: whether it's what we eat, or how we move, or when we take some time out for ourselves. When we're able to balance our mood through the small things, we're far better placed to access a state of what I call 'everyday happiness', rather than pinning all our hope (and happiness) on a particular event, outcome or person.

And in the same way that we can control how the small things in our day go, we can also control how we *feel* about them. I always come back to that old adage: 'This too shall pass.' If you had a bad time, this too shall pass. If you had a good time, this too shall pass. That's a fact of life. For me, that's the secret to getting your mind in a better place. It's also knowing that wherever you are on that cycle (good, indifferent or bad), the one constant is the presence of the small things. Appreciating the seasons (whether that's sunshine and sunny mornings, or even the freshness of rain), Sunday lie-ins, a cup of tea with a good friend, the hobbies that you love and can do for not much cost or effort, walking your dog in the park, treating yourself to a nice bunch of flowers. The impact of paying attention to the little things as much as the big things is threefold. It makes you stronger for the tough times, keeps your feet grounded for the good times and makes you appreciate life more.

ENJOY the little things

KEEP IT REAL

Although I have achieved a certain level of success, my happiness markers have stayed pretty constant throughout my life. I do like to treat myself to a nice bag or coat once in a while, but the things that made me happy twenty years ago are the same things that make me happy today. Fresh air, horse riding, running a nice bath, an early night, having a laugh with good friends, discovering a great author and enjoying their latest book. I also think it's about drawing a line between happiness and what you could call moments of extravagant joy. It's great fun going to a party in a new dress or going on a luxury holiday. But equally, the smaller, seemingly mundane stuff will also give you something back. It's about filling both buckets – have the moments of crazy fun but prioritize and take pleasure in the little moments.

EVERYTHING IS FIXABLE

I was totally unprepared for building my company NEOM in many ways and it's been a really steep learning curve. But whenever I've been faced with challenges, I've tried to see them as a problem to get around, rather than something that's going to stop me in my tracks. Broadly speaking, most things are fix-able. It might not be in the way that you would hope, and you might not have option A, B or even option C, but it is all fixable. Having that mindset has definitely helped me with building a business and made me not take things so seriously, which means I've enjoyed it more along the way and been able to keep my head up and my mood high.

VALUE YOUR VALUES

Values are a really important piece in the happiness jigsaw, but I think we can sometimes overlook them in the pursuit of the other things we think will make us happy in the short term. A career coach once told me to spend a bit of time working out my own values, because it's a really great way of figuring yourself out. I've always found that really helpful – I think you can only be truly happy if you're living your authentic life. Some of my core values are having fun in whatever I'm doing, friends, learn-ing and growth, creativity, authenticity and strength. That's not to say my values are universal for everyone, but they're right for me. Rather than chasing or wanting something because I think it will make me happy, I make sure those values show up in what-ever I'm doing. And inevitably, happiness happens along the way. You don't think about it because you're doing it.

WHY NOT TRY . . . A VALUE AUDIT

Think about what your personal values are. Have you done something that aligns to those personal values this week, this month or this year? Make it very specific to you. Write down as many as you want, and then spend a week figuring out what five resonate most with you and then, how you can implement them. Our values can show up in our jobs, our relationships, our choices, how we spend our free time and how we treat ourselves. Maybe your values are already aligned and this is just another happiness reminder for you. Remember, there's no better or worse values, they're the ones that feel right for you.

SMALL STEPS TO HAPPINESS

So, happiness doesn't have to always mean something big or exciting, and it's something that each of us has control over. This sounds great in theory, but how exactly do we improve our mood and happiness levels? In his book *Happy Mind, Happy Life,* Dr Rangan Chatterjee coined the term 'junk happiness' and talked about how we often fill ourselves up with things that bring us instant gratification but ultimately don't last, instead of prioritizing what he calls our 'core happiness', which is based around contentment, feeling in control and in alignment with who we really are.

I absolutely agree with this concept. What we feed ourselves is really important and I'm not just talking from a nutritional point of view. It's the company we keep, the news we engage with, the thoughts that we tell ourselves in our heads. By actively choosing to nourish ourselves with positive things, we have control over our mood in that moment and, ultimately, over our long-term happiness.

When I first planned this chapter, it seemed logical to look at all the external things we can change in our life first. But then I thought, unless we have our mindset right, there's a good chance we won't get the most out of what we do, or even know why we're doing it in the first place. So let's go inward and start with the concept of neuroplasticity.

THE NEW SCIENCE BEHIND HAPPINESS

Neuroplasticity is a hot topic; it refers to the brain's ability to change and grow throughout our lives. Our brains are made up of neural pathways, which send signals from one part of our brain to the other. Rather than being biologically fixed, neural pathways are more like patterns that have been learned over time. I think it's helpful to think of the brain like a map: some routes are more trodden than others. When we think of something, our neural pathways are 'fired and wired' to form a certain response in our brain. The next time we think of that same thing, the same pattern lights up again and again . . . The result is that our brains become fixed to that certain pattern, whether it's good or bad.

'We have the ability to rewire our brains through neuroplasticity.'

Positive neuroplasticity occurs as a result of new learnings, experiences and memory formations, which causes new neural pathways to strengthen. This can be anything from starting a new form of exercise or hobby, learning a language, taking up a creative pursuit like writing or even going travelling. With the right training or therapy, it can be possible for us to unlearn unhelpful thought patterns or automatic stress responses and carve out new response routes that make us more robust, positive and resilient. While neuroplasticity is clearly a very complex area and depends on individual circumstances, there are basic learnings that we can all apply to our own lives. Trying something new or challenging has proven benefits for the brain and neuroplasticity can help us become happier at any age.

EPIGENETICS

Epigenetics is another emerging area of scientific research that shows how environmental influences and lifestyle factors can affect the way we express our genes. Scientists have found that our genes aren't always set in stone to be passed from generation to generation. Regardless of our family history and traits, things like childhood experiences and the quality of our nutrition, our stress levels, physical exercise and working habits have the potential to change not only our emotional temperament and physical health, but that of our children, too. Happiness can be right here in front of us and is something much more practical and achievable than we perhaps realized before.

How to train your brain

* Pick one activity and stick to it. It's not just what you do, but the consistency and commitment to improve.
* Sign up to a class. Classes are a good way to learn specific skills, like painting, pottery or a new language. The social aspect and paying for a chunk of classes in advance will help to keep you committed.
* Set a practice schedule that fits around the rest of your commitments so you're more likely to keep on track and not resent missing out on other things.

ATTITUDE

Positive psychology is a relatively new branch of psychology and is a scientific approach to studying human thoughts, feelings, and behaviour, with a focus on strengths instead of weaknesses, and building the good in life instead of repairing the bad. It explores how meaning, pleasure, creativity, good relationships and accomplishments are all important factors in our mental health and advocates that focusing on strengthening these will help people flourish and live their best lives. This idea of focusing on the positives is music to my ears.

Of course, some people may find they take happiness from certain things more than others. For example, creativity is an absolute must for me. I now know myself well enough to ensure I have a creative outlet – whether that's creating a new Pinterest mood board at work for a new campaign or cooking up a new recipe for a group of friends on a Thursday night. It's imperative for me and a huge factor in how content I feel.

Vanessa King is a Positive Psychology Expert for Action for Happiness and the author of *How to be Happy: 10 Keys to Happier Living*. 'It's true that some of us are naturally more hopeful or optimistic than others,' she says. 'There's also evidence that we can learn to become more hopeful and optimistic. We know from the research that when people have what's called "realistic optimism", which means generally expecting things to turn out reasonably well, it tends to have lots of positive ramifications for all sorts of things such as for our wellbeing, relationships and performance.'

'Optimistic explanatory style is a way of thinking identified by cognitive psychologists,' says Vanessa. 'People who have this optimistic style tend to believe that when things go wrong it's generally not only their fault and not something that's going to pervade other aspects of their life or be permanent. Clearly, many factors like our environment and circumstances have an impact on us, not all of which we can change, but psychologists and neuro-scientists have shown that we can learn new skills and habits of mind that can contribute to feeling happier. The brain can change with intention and practice. It doesn't mean you might go from being the deepest pessimist through to the complete opposite. But you can certainly move in the right direction and in constructive ways that are likely to serve you better psychologically.'

GRATITUDE

As I touched on earlier, an effective way of improving your mood/happiness is practising gratitude: taking a moment each day to reflect on what you are thankful for, what has gone well or is making you happy. Research has found that a daily writing practice like this can make people feel more optimistic about their lives and even result in fewer visits to the doctor. One study found that healthcare workers who kept a gratitude diary showed a 28 per cent reduction in stress levels, while another study asked participants to write and personally deliver a letter to someone they'd never thanked properly for their kindness. Participants reported a big increase in happiness scores, with the results lasting for up to a month.

In the chapter on Stress I spoke about how I write down three good things that happened that day every night before I go to bed. It's such a simple thing but it can flick the switch in my mind from negative to positive and remind me that even on the trying days, things weren't completely terrible. Life can feel so busy and we're often on to the next thing and can forget all the good things that happened: a meeting or work call that went well, a walk in the sun-shine or a nice message from a friend you haven't heard from in a while. Keeping a list restores a sense of 'all is well' in me, and I go off to sleep in a much better state of mind. Plus, writing things down in a specific notebook means I can always look back through it and remind myself of the good stuff. This is a process wellbeing expert and Yale Professor Laurie Santos calls 'tracking' your happiness.

TAKE A MOMENT

What gratitude practice can you bring into your life? It could be keeping a daily list, writing someone a letter (and delivering it in person) or savouring and recording the little moments, like enjoying a good coffee.

'HAPPINESS IS A CONSCIOUS CHOICE'

Mo Gawdat, bestselling author of *Solve for Happy*, is a remarkable person and someone who I've been lucky enough to have on my podcast, *The NEOM No BS Guide to Wellbeing*. Mo was the former Chief Business Officer at Google who spent over a decade engineering an equation for happiness as the blueprint for a more meaningful life. As an engineer, Mo believed that everything has an equation and Mo's own method was put to the test when his son Ali suddenly died at the age of twenty-one. By using his own happiness equation, Mo has not only managed to survive the unimaginable loss that he and his family have been through, but is able to now live in a state of peace, contentment and even joy. Mo's happiness equation boils down to one simple formula: 'If you perceive the events as equal or greater than your expectations, you're happy – or at least not unhappy.'

The key to experiencing true, long-lasting happiness is to reframe how we expect to experience it. Mo says that happiness is the 'absence of unhappiness' and is our default state; so we don't need to wait for our next holiday, it can be found in the here and now. It might sound easier said than done when you're at a low ebb or have had a string of bad luck, but mindset is key; happiness is in our own hands and each of us makes the conscious choice to be happy (or unhappy). Having suffered with the unimaginable pain of losing a child, Mo's advice on how we can all influence our happiness is an invaluable lesson for us all to learn. This starts with not automatically believing our negative thoughts, which are a hangover from our ancient brains that were wired to be vigilant by constantly looking out for threats. Thousands of years later, our brains still default to this primitive pattern (and hence why we're more likely to be drawn to bad news). 'A thought can take its thinker through years of suffering,' Mo says. 'Happiness depends entirely on how we control every thought.'

> **'Do your best at whatever you're doing now.
> This is the moment, the only one you can count on.
> Live in it fully, and the rest will take care of itself.'**

I absolutely love Mo's happiness equation and how it's about learning to roll with the punches and having a steady equilibrium, instead of always living in the highs and lows. *Solve for Happy* is a brilliant and inspirational read and I recommend it to anyone looking for more joy, meaning and sunshine in their lives, no matter their circumstances.

HOPE THEORY

Another helpful theory that I came across recently when researching innovative ways of thinking about our happiness was devised by positive psychologist Charles Snyder. Hope theory is made up of three key elements: goals (thinking in a goal-oriented way), pathways (finding ways to achieve your goals) and agency (believing that you can instigate change).

'In psychology, hope theory is more than our common use of the word *hope*,' says Vanessa King. 'It offers a practical framework for moving forward. Starting from where you are at, it involves asking yourself: what do you realistically hope for and are most motivated towards? Then, what are the pathways you can take towards that? Then, what obstacles are you likely to encounter and how might you get round them? It creates a sense of agency, rather than feeling things are hopeless, meaning you're much more likely to do what you can. Even in tough times it can help us look for small glimmers of hope and nudges forward.'

I really like the idea of hope theory because it encapsulates a lot of what we have covered in this chapter. The idea that we have agency over our own happiness, that things are never normally as bad or unfixable as we might imagine them to be and that no matter what we encounter, if we keep the right mindset and have enough resilience, good things will always come our way again.

Try hope theory for yourself:

1. What do you realistically hope for? Why?

2. What steps can you take to get there?

3. What might get in your way and how will you get round them?

It's a bad day
NOT a bad life

KEEP LEARNING

A growth mindset is the belief that we can develop our skills and talents through learning, hard work and the right strategies, as well as seeing failure as an opportunity for growth. A fixed mindset on the other hand means that we believe that our intelligence or ability is fixed at a certain level, and that if we're not good at something, we'll never improve. I think it's fairly clear, therefore, that having a growth mindset as opposed to a fixed mindset can massively determine how we engage with life. I think it can mean that we also have a certain view of the world, or other people, and we act on assumptions rather than real knowledge or experience, which can leave us in a rather small and fearful place. But as we've discussed, we weren't born with our current mindset and the discovery of neuroplasticity is evidence that we can change our negative thought patterns through learning and development.

Personally, I've always loved learning new things. For me, constantly trying to grow in areas that we're interested in means we just get the best out of life. I always say building NEOM was like climbing Mount Everest in flip flops. I couldn't have done it without a growth mindset, and I've been constantly learning – and failing – along the way. Something that doesn't work out isn't an ending. It just means taking a different route and – more often than not – you end up with an even better solution. For me, this was building a company but it will be different for you. It could be learning a new skill, starting a side hustle, changing jobs or just looking at new ways to solve problems. Developing in different areas of your life will increase your confidence and capabilities and, in turn, your happiness. What new thing can you start today, or what different approach can you take to something? Surprise yourself! You never know, you might have a secret talent or skill ready to be unlocked.

Ask me anything

Q: Do you believe in mantras and do you use them?
A: I'm not big on mantras because sometimes they sound a bit too worthy for me. But I do like 'Today I will have a good day because it's my choice.'

THE POWER OF FIRSTS

People are generally happier with their lives if they hold positive nostalgic views of the past, says Meik Wiking, founder of the Happiness Research Institute in Copenhagen. In his book *Happy Moments*, Meik talks about how nostalgia can help to boost our self-esteem and the feeling of being loved and appreciated by others. 'This means that long-term happiness can depend on your ability to form a positive memory of the past,' he writes.

Many of the most potent positive memories are associated with new or novel experiences, such as our first kiss, first love, the first time we went travelling or got our first car, the first time we saw someone in concert who we loved. Unsurprisingly, most of our memories are between the age of fifteen and thirty, while the Happiness Research Institute found that nearly a quarter of people's memories were of novel or extraordinary experiences. We can still have new experiences as we get older, but by harnessing the power of firsts, we're more likely to pay the feel-good factor forward (as well as enjoying ourselves at the time).

Interestingly, we're also more likely to enjoy the music that we liked as adolescents, as this was a time of firsts. Music can make us travel to a happy memory: 'One note and we're taken back to that time, that place, that mood,' says Wiking.

MAKE SOME NEW FIRSTS

When was the last time you tried something new, or did something different? Try adding in some 'firsts' on a regular basis – even something as small as going on a new walk – and see if it has an impact on your mood. Alternatively, create a happy playlist of all those classic tunes from your youth that you still remember all the words to and channel your inner teen. It might even give you plenty to write about in your gratitude journal – double-win!

FIND YOUR FLOW

The 'Flow' state is a term coined by the Hungarian psychologist Mihaly Csikszentmihalyi and describes a state of concentration so focused that a person becomes completely absorbed in an activity. Csikszentmihalyi has called it the 'secret to happiness' and flow has been linked to lower stress and anxiety, as well as building resilience in adverse situations, by distracting the brain away from self-focus and negative thought patterns.

In theory, flow occurs when the level of skill matches the challenge (meaning you can successfully do the thing that you're doing), but I don't think you have to get too prescriptive about what that looks like. One place I can quite easily get into flow is the middle part of exercise (once I've got past the warm-up and hard bit). I also enjoy my work, so I get into a flow doing something like working up new creative concepts for our store window designs or formulating new NEOM product ideas with our product development team. You don't have to necessarily go and do a 'thing'. I know when I'm in my flow when a) time goes by quickly and b) I feel energized and a sense of achievement afterwards.

'Procrastination can be the enemy of happiness. Done is always better than perfect.'

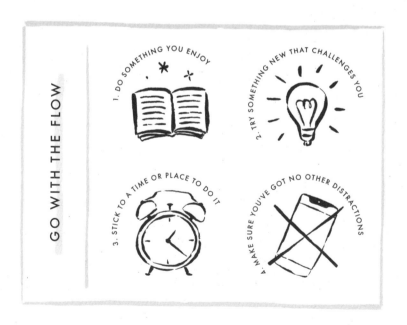

GO WITH THE FLOW

1. DO SOMETHING YOU ENJOY

2. TRY SOMETHING NEW THAT CHALLENGES YOU

3. STICK TO A TIME OR PLACE TO DO IT

4. MAKE SURE YOU'VE GOT NO OTHER DISTRACTIONS

RESILIENCE AND 'ORDINARY MAGIC'

Resilience is an interesting one for me in the context of happiness because I think, as a mum, it can be in our nature to remove difficulty or find a distraction when our kids get upset about something, rather than letting them sit with an emotion or navigate a tricky situation. But if we (and they) learn to roll with the punches we're better equipped to take things on the next time they come round. 'The keys to happier living are also the keys to resilience,' says positive psychology expert Vanessa King. 'It's not about doing certain things and as a result expecting we're going to be happy forever after, because life's not like that. It has ups and downs. Resilience helps us cope when times are tough and a lot of that is around our habits of thinking. It also includes self-care and seeking help when we need it. Importantly, seeking help is not a sign of weakness. It's a sign of strength. We are more resilient when we have support from others.'

'Ordinary magic' is a phrase coined by an American psychologist called Ann Masten. 'In terms of human evolution, every single one of us comes from a long line of people who've survived all sorts of things over millennia,' says Vanessa. 'It doesn't always feel like it, but we are a resilient species – we keep going and finding ways to adapt. Day-to-day, things don't always work out how we planned but we can find ways to get around or overcome obstacles and issues. This can help put things in perspective. We could be dealing with a disappointment that feels really hard and painful at the time, but we can ask ourselves if this thing that is worrying or upsetting me now, will it still feel as painful and as big a deal in a year or ten years' time? It probably won't. That's ordinary magic and we all have it.'

SELF-ACCEPTANCE VS SELF ESTEEM

Fundamentally, I believe our own happiness comes down to how we treat ourselves. Chartered psychologist Suzy Reading talks about the importance of self-compassion on page 88, and my own mantra is talking to myself the way I would to a good friend, or my younger self. Having that kindly inner dialogue and not being hard on ourselves is key, and similarly there's something important to be said about self-acceptance.

'Self-esteem tends to be about comparing ourselves to others and feeling better or worse than them. In contrast, self-acceptance is knowing our strengths and weaknesses and accepting we don't need to be perfect – and that no one is perfect, either,' says Vanessa King. 'We don't need to feel better than other people in order to feel good.'

We tend to become a bit more accepting of ourselves with age and wisdom, but we can start to practise self-acceptance at any time. 'We can start by noticing the things we do right, however small. This helps us start to identify our strengths and things that we naturally do well and we find energizing,' Vanessa says. 'This can be hard at first as naturally we focus on all the things we think we do wrong. Also, sometimes it's actually quite hard to notice our strengths, because things feel very natural to us, but it's interesting to see what other people see in us. It's really quite important to get to know ourselves and see our good bits as well as what we'd like to get better at.'

TAKE A MOMENT

If you find it difficult to recognize your strengths and skills, ask a trusted other or someone who you respect to list five things they like about you. Get comfortable with owning them and see where you can let them show up more in your life.

REDEFINING SUCCESS

Another part of Mo Gawdat's perspective on happiness is that success doesn't always guarantee happiness. I think there's huge importance in remembering that. When we think about success, more often than not we associate it with careers, status, material possessions and how much is in the bank.

Of course, we all want financial security and recognition and it's good to have nice things. A career is important and can give us a sense of purpose. But the bottom line is that if we're working 60 hours a week in a job that doesn't fulfil us and we're hardly ever seeing friends or family or having any downtime, chances are that we're not going to be very happy.

Redefining success means taking a bit of time out to think about it. Is what we're striving for or holding on to *really* making us happy? As with wellbeing, I think it's helpful to define those things into pillars. The point of success is working out what 'good' looks like to you. And then breaking this down into little bits so you can start to build on them.

> '**Success is loving life and daring to lead it.**'
>
> – Maya Angelou

THE CYCLE OF KINDNESS: PASS IT ON

Another insight that I have found incredibly helpful is that doing good for others works both ways, as performing small acts of kindness produces endorphins, also known as the 'helper's high'. Studies say this activates the reward centre in our brain, which means we're more likely to do it again, ingraining those positive actions. People who help others report lower levels of stress, while a 2013 study found a link between volunteering and reduced blood pressure. Doing good at work also makes us happier; apparently, people who are considered altruists in the workplace are more committed to their jobs and are less likely to leave, while a University of Wisconsin study found that individuals in their mid-thirties who rated helping others in their work as important reported they were happier with their life when surveyed thirty years later.

There's so much great data on the science of giving but what I think this all illustrates is how helping others isn't just a one-off act. It can have a cumulative effect on our happiness, and therefore our wellbeing. Professor Laurie Santos ran Yale's most subscribed course, The Science of Well-Being. 'Research shows that we are happiest when we're doing for other people,' she says. 'The research so far shows that the actions that we do for other people can have relatively long-standing happiness effects. They're the kind of things that can boost your wellbeing, even when you think back on them.'

Leading happiness researcher Sonja Lyubomirsky has found that performing positive acts once a week led to the most happiness. This doesn't mean we all have to engage Mother Theresa levels of selflessness or spend our days doing good deeds. Texting a friend when you remember they've had a tough meeting or on a special anniversary can count!

'People who engage in kind acts
become happier over time.'

– Sonja Lyubomirsky, author of *The How of Happiness*.

SLEEP

As I've said throughout these pages, I think of sleep as the key to every aspect of our wellbeing and, particularly when it comes to mood, sleep is the one place where we can make the biggest difference, with the least amount of effort. If you've zoomed past Chapter 1 and straight to this section, The 11 Golden Rules for Better Sleep on page 45 is a brilliant blueprint for helping to keep your mood in a more balanced state. We all know we feel our best with enough sleep and vice versa – this is just a reminder that it's within our power to change that.

When it comes to the impact of sleep on our mood, it isn't surprising to learn that studies consistently show that sleep deprivation can cause fatigue, irritability and reduced attention, as well as negatively impact our mental health; even partial sleep deprivation can have an impact on mood. A 2019 Iowa State University study found that after two nights of sleep restriction, people were more reactive to noise in their surroundings, and less able to concentrate on tasks. While the average amount of sleep a person needs can depend on things like physiology and age, research shows the body's ability to function declines if sleep isn't in the 7- to 8-hour range.

When we have slept badly we also tend to eat less healthily. Leptin and ghrelin are the 'hunger hormones' that are integral to our appetite and energy management. Leptin is the satiety or full-ness hormone, while ghrelin is the hormone that makes us feel hungry. When we're sleep-deprived, our levels of leptin decrease while our levels of ghrelin go up, making us feel hungrier, with studies showing that we're more likely to reach for calorie-dense, fatty foods, which can have an impact on our mood.

GOOD MOOD FOOD

We've covered the nutritional fundamentals in the Stress chapter but it goes without saying that what we eat has a massive impact on how we feel. Tryptophan-rich foods are key; this amino acid is important for serotonin production and as we can't make it ourselves we have to get it from our diet. It's found in chicken and turkey, whole milk, whole oats, nuts and seeds, eggs, salmon, fruits like pineapple, bananas, kiwi fruit and tomatoes, green leafy veg like spinach, broccoli and watercress, yogurt and chickpeas.

Omega 3 is essential for our brains (see page 197), for brain development and brain health throughout our life, with studies showing it can be beneficial for treating depression. Just like tryptophan, our bodies can't make it by itself, so we need to get it from other sources. EPA and DHA are two essential fatty acids crucial for brain health and they're found almost exclusively in oily fish and seafood, like sardines and mackerel, while ALA is another type of plant-based fatty acid and can be found in things like soya beans, flaxseeds and nuts.

Don't forget the B vitamins: B12 and B6 play a vital role in our psychological wellbeing and help regulate levels of serotonin and dopamine. B12 is mainly found in animal-derived products like lean meat, dairy and eggs as well as yeast extracts and B12 breakfast cereals. Good sources of B6 include chicken and turkey, peanuts, soya beans, wheatgerm, oats, bananas, milk and low-sugar fortified breakfast cereals. (For a deeper dive into how B vitamins work, turn to page 102.)

THE HAPPINESS ECONOMY

The saying goes we are what we eat, but we're also an accumulation of the people we surround ourselves with. While the number of friends we need differs from person to person, and that number changes over our lifetime, choosing uplifting company appears to be the one defining payback when it comes to long-term happiness. What's more, happiness appears to be contagious. An influential US study looking at 5,000 people over a twenty-year period found that the happiness of an individual was associated with the happiness of people up to three degrees removed from their immediate social network. In other words, you're more likely to be happy if your friend's friend is happy.

While researchers concluded that physical proximity played a significant factor (as in meeting up in real life rather than just being Facebook friends), it seems that happiness can belong to a larger group of people rather than just being an individual experience. Think of it a bit like a happiness economy: choosing to surround yourself with positive people isn't just good for you and the people you directly interact with, it can also pay your happiness forward.

CAN WE CATCH A BAD MOOD?

If happiness is infectious, does the same apply to unhappiness? Yes, according to research from Oxford and Birmingham universities. The small-scale study of seventy-nine teenagers found that respondents matched their mood when interacting with gloomier individuals, with researchers concluding that bad moods were more contagious than good ones. While it might come as little surprise for this particular teenage demographic (we've all been there), it would appear that you can catch a bad mood at any age. Studies show that rude people tend to cluster in groups, while emotional contagion can spread through workplaces.

Be the
ENERGY
you want
to attract

POSITIVE WAYS TO USE SOCIAL MEDIA

Social media gets a bad rap when it comes to the negative mental health effects, but there are still lots of benefits. Again, it's how you use it and how much time you spend on there. Dedicate an hour or some proper time to curate your news feed or timeline and only follow accounts that you find interesting, useful, relevant and inspiring. People who actively engage with others' posts such as commenting and sharing also report higher levels of social wellbeing and satisfaction than those who scroll passively. Or why not try a social media sabbatical? A 2022 Bath University study found that participants who took a one-week break

reported improved mood and less overall anxiety, with researchers concluding that even just a small break can have an impact.

NO NEWS IS GOOD NEWS

Before rolling news coverage, we used to get our news twice a
day with a morning newspaper and evening TV bulletin. Now it
runs through constantly in a variety of different ways. On average, people in the UK check their smartphones every 12 minutes
of the waking day, according to a 2021 Ofcom survey, with 40
per cent of adults checking their phone within 5 minutes of
waking up.

It's not just how much we look at the news, but how we consume it. Another 2021 survey found that at least 71 per cent of
American adults used social media as a go-to news source. Meanwhile in 2022 TikTok was the fastest growing news source in the
UK for people aged sixteen to twenty-four. According to another
2022 global survey looking at social media trust and consumption, large proportions of people say they do not trust social media
as news sources but still access the networks on a daily basis.

Bad news sells, or at least gets shared more. We have an
inbuilt negativity bias (more on that in a bit) and studies show
that we're more likely to click on a headline containing negative
words than positive ones. Bad news also outweighs the good: a
2019 study across six different countries found that the negative
news made up 85 per cent of news output. The UK and the
Netherlands were most likely to report negative news, with only
14 per cent of UK news coverage being positive.

The fact that most news feels bad probably isn't news to us.
But engaging with negative news can affect us more than we
think. 'Doomscrolling' was named Oxford Dictionary's word of

the year in 2020 and has been linked to increased levels of anxiety and negative mood.

There's also some interesting research on how being exposed to negative news can make our own problems feel worse. A study published in the *British Journal of Psychology* investigated the physiological impact of TV news bulletins. Three groups were shown 14-minute TV news bulletins that were edited to display either positive, neutral or negative news content material. Participants who watched the negative bulletins showed an increase in both anxious and sad moods, as well as a significant increase in the tendency to catastrophize a personal worry. It doesn't even matter if the news doesn't directly affect us. Researchers also suggest that negatively themed TV news programmes can 'exacerbate a range of personal concerns that are not specifically relevant to the content of the programme'. Bad news can feel like it's everywhere but the science shows that it's disproportionate and not always an accurate representation of reality, especially in our own here and now.

That's interesting
British people spend the equivalent of scrolling three times the height of the Eiffel Tower every day. This is according to a survey of 1,000 people from online optical retailer Lenstore.

START A HAPPY NEWS HABIT

Why not try starting the day with some good news, or swap a scroll on social media for a positive new site instead? Here are some of my favourites:

Positive News (www.positive.news)
Good News Network (www.goodnewsnetwork.org)
The Happy Newspaper (www.thehappynewspaper.com)

NATURE AND HAPPINESS

As with the other pillars of our wellbeing, the outdoors also has a direct impact on our mood. We feel it instinctively when the sun is shining down on us, or we can smell freshly cut grass, and there's just a huge amount of evidence on the mood-boosting benefits of being out in nature. A University of Washington study found that time in nature is associated with an increase in: 'happiness, subjective wellbeing, positive social interactions and a sense of purpose and meaning in life'. Being out in nature can make us nicer as well: another series of Canadian studies found that exposure to nature (as opposed to a more urban environment) makes us more likely to cooperate with others, as well as be more friendly to people, both ones we know and strangers.

Time in nature can also make us more creative. Nature can induce in us a sense of awe, researchers say, which is linked to more expansive thinking, as well as making us more hopeful by shifting our sense of time, away from deadlines and the everyday. Got things on your mind? Get into some green. Studies say immersion in a physically large expanse of nature can induce a mentally bigger perspective and make us worry less about our problems.

LIVING WALLS

Biophilia is the belief that humans have a genetic tendency to seek connections with nature, since our ancestors evolved in

5 EASY WAYS
TO BRING BIOPHILIA INTO
YOUR HOME OR OFFICE

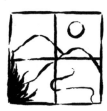

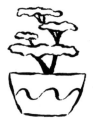

1. MAKE THE MOST OF NATURAL LIGHT.
STUDIES SHOW THAT WORKING BY
A WINDOW MAKES US FEEL HAPPIER
AND ENERGIZED.

2. ADD SOME GREENERY.
PUT A PLANT ON YOUR DESK, ADD A HERB
GARDEN TO YOUR KITCHEN WINDOW OR
HANG A TRAILING PLANT FROM THE CEILING
IF YOU'RE SHORT ON SPACE.

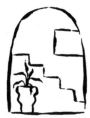

**3. WARM UP INSIDE SPACES
WITH NATURAL COLOURS
AND TEXTILES.**

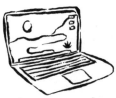

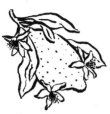

4. GREEN UP YOUR TECH.
STUDIES SHOW THAT NATURE
BASED SCREENSAVERS AND VIRTUAL
BACKGROUNDS CAN BOOST CREATIVITY
AND REDUCE STRESS.

**5. INDULGE YOUR SENSES
WITH NEOM'S SCENT TO
MAKE YOU HAPPY RANGE.**
REFRESHING, FLORAL NEROLI IS SWEETENED
BY FRUITY MIMOSA AND A PURELY POSITIVE
LIFT OF INVIGORATING SICILIAN LEMON.
INVOKE THE FEELING OF SUMMER MORNINGS
AND THE SMELL OF FRESHLY CUT GRASS
IN THE AIR = PURE HAPPY VIBES!

233

wild settings and relied on the environment for survival. Bio-philic design is the practice of bringing nature into our built environments and includes things like natural daylight and ven-tilation (sunny spots and fresh air), natural colours and textures, plants, water features and animals (think bringing your dog to the office rather than a herd of rampaging cows). Biophilic office design has been linked to higher levels of productivity and happiness and has even boosted immune health.

GOOD MOVES

When it comes to feeling better, movement shouldn't just be functional but should be something that brings us a bit of joy. A great way to inject a bit of fun into your exercise is to do it with someone else, or a group of people. Studies show that the social benefits of shared exercise include improved communication skills, higher levels of motivation and happiness and better self-esteem. Joining a netball team not your bag? Try combining movement with a social activity instead, like catching up over a hike at the weekend rather than dinner, or tie it in with vol-unteering for a double hit of exercise endorphins and the 'helper's high' associated with altruistic acts. For example, Good Gym is a charity of runners, walkers and cyclists who combine exercise with helping communities – why not see if they oper-ate near you?

A CASCADE OF POSITIVE EVENTS

What's really interesting is that not only can exercise make you feel good in the moment, it can also keep you feeling better for longer than you even realize. A US study found that people who exercised reported more positive social interactions with friends and family on that day, with researchers concluding that the feel-good effects we get from exercise can 'cascade' into another positive event such as a subsequent good interaction, or a small act that brings someone else happiness. Another 2010 study found that even brief, low-intensity episodes of physical activity such as walking can result in significant same-day mood improvements. So, by investing some time in movement earlier in the day, you really are setting yourself up for a more positive day.

REFRAMING REST AS REJUVENATION

Rest can feel like a bit of a lost art these days and more often than not, we just don't make time for it (or think we have the time). Guilt about doing 'nothing' is one of the biggest blockers, but the science shows that prioritizing rest makes us happier and more productive. 'I think that describing rest as a nourishing act that brings you back to balance can be really helpful in the context of mood,' says Suzy Reading. 'Rest needn't be lying down in stillness, doing nothing, on your own. It can be something gently invigorating like joyful movement, a creative pursuit or connecting with a kindred spirit. Ask yourself, what will help you feel a greater sense of harmony and peace? This is rest.' Still struggle to switch off? 'If the word rest itself feels laden with negative association, call it rejuvenation and feel the freedom this facilitates,' says Suzy.

I am in charge
of how I feel
today and I
am choosing
HAPPINESS

FINAL THOUGHTS

As I said at the start, this pillar is perhaps the hardest to define in many ways, because the idea of 'happiness' is so subjective. But I hope that recognizing happiness is something that we do have material control over has inspired you and, well, made you happier! Being in a good mood is not some magical concept and there is now amazing research to show that we can actually make our brains healthier, just as we can with the rest of our body, from what we put in, to what we choose to leave out. So, what will you choose to put in and leave out?

I grew up thinking happiness was a destination – having the big house, the successful business, that amazing beach holiday, but the one thing I've realized over the last twenty years of my career in this industry is that practising gratitude and appreciating the little things in my everyday life trumps anything I could buy or obtain. Our mantra at NEOM has always been 'small steps, big difference' and I swear by my gratitude diary at night before I go to bed – just a moment to reflect on all the little things that have gone right that day – a phone call with a friend that made me laugh, the sweet peas finally starting to bloom, an unexpected sunny afternoon, burning our Happiness Fragrance with a glass of wine at sunset, my teenager being in a good mood . . . these are the good things in life for me, and reflecting on them can make me feel noticeably happier. If there's one thing I'd like you to take away from this chapter, I'd say it's this question: what are your small steps to happiness?

CONCLUSION

I've loved putting *The Four Ways to Wellbeing* together and I really hope you've enjoyed the book, and have found it useful. I think the best advice I can give here is this: when it comes to creating your own personal toolkit, make it something that *you* like. You're well versed with the four pillars of wellbeing now but play around with what suits you. It is going to be trial and error and it will take time, so you should enjoy doing it. Also, remember that it will always be a work in progress. Our wellbeing needs are going to change – as we grow older, through the seasons, as our hormones change, through different life circumstances . . . The secret is to be invested enough in your own wellbeing to keep trying new things and seeing what works.

Recommendation is key in the wellbeing space, so I've put together a list of all the books, people and brands that I really rate, who are driving the new science and pushing the boundaries in coming up with exciting concepts. This is my own Little Black Book of Wellbeing contacts, but I definitely recommend that you get together a list of brands that you trust and that you've done your research on. I always love hearing from people in the wellbeing community and sharing knowledge, so get in touch with your own tips and recommendations.

Enjoy building your wellbeing toolkit! Why not listen to more experts over on my podcast, *The NEOM No BS Guide to Wellbeing*. You can also find out more about NEOM by scanning the QR code below.

@nicolaelliottneom

NICOLA'S LITTLE BLACK
BOOK OF WELLBEING

The brilliant experts who have contributed to my book

Nick Witton

Sleep specialist and performance coach
elite-sleep.co.uk
@nick_elitesleep

Richie Norton

Wellbeing and performance coach and author of *Lift Your Vibe*
thestrengthtemple.com
@richienorton

Alice Mackintosh

Registered nutritional therapist and co-author of *The Happy Kitchen: Good Mood Food*
alicemackintosh.com | equilondon.com
@alicemackintosh_nutrition

Suzy Reading
Chartered psychologist and author of *Rest to Reset* and *Self-Care for Tough Times*
suzyreading.co.uk
@suzyreading

James Rafael
Yoga and mindfulness teacher
jamesrafael.com
@jamesyoga

Professor Annice Mukherjee
Doctor, hormone specialist and author of *The Complete Guide to the Menopause*
hormonewise.co.uk
@the.hormone.doc

Dr Deepak Ravindran
Pain management specialist and author of *The Pain-Free Mindset*
deepakravindran.co.uk
@drdeepakravindran

Eve Kalinik
Nutritional therapist and author of *Be Good to Your Gut* and *Happy Gut, Happy Mind*
evekalinik.com
@evekalinik

Deirdre Egan

Nutritionist and hormonal health coach

deirdreegan.com

@deirdreegannutrition

Joshua Fletcher

Psychotherapist and author of *Untangle Your Anxiety, Anxiety: Panicking About Panic* and *Anxiety: Practical About Panic*

schoolofanxiety.com

The Panic Pod podcast

@anxietyjosh

Stuart Sandeman

Breath coach and author of *Breathe In, Breathe Out*

breathpod.com

@breathpod

Dr Jenna Macciochi

Immunologist and author of *Immunity: The Science of Staying Well* and *Your Blueprint for Strong Immunity*

drjennamacciochi.com

@dr_jenna_macciochi

Vanessa King

Leading expert on the practical application of the science of happiness, resilience and wellbeing and author of *How to be Happy: 10 Keys to Happier Living*

thechangespace.com

Board Member for Action for Happiness

actionforhappiness.org

Wellbeing thought leaders and websites

Susannah Taylor
Fabulous wellbeing journalist
@susannahtaylor_

Hip and healthy
Great online magazine for the latest wellbeing news
hipandhealthy.com

Tiny Buddha
Tinybuddha.com

Well + Good
wellandgood.com
@iamwellandgood

Other experts and authors

Dr Martha Deiros Collado
Clinical psychologist
drmarthapsychologist.com
@dr.martha.psychologist

Chloe Brotheridge
Anxiety hypnotherapist and coach and author of
The Anxiety Solution
@chloebrotheridge

Dr Will Cole
Leading functional medicine expert and author of *Gut Feelings*,
Intuitive Fasting and *The Inflammation Spectrum*
@drwillcole

Kathryn Pinkham
Sleep and insomnia specialist
theinsomniaclinic.co.uk
@theinsomniaclinic

Dr Julie Smith
Clinical psychologist and author of *Why Has Nobody Told Me
This Before?*
@drjuliesmith

Tony Schwartz
Author of *The Way We're Working Isn't Working*

Dr Zoe Williams
NHS GP
@drzoewilliams

Dr Mariel Buqué
Psychologist and author of *Break the Cycle*
drmarielbuque.com
@dr.marielbuque

Dr Emma Hepburn
Clinical psychologist and author of *A Toolkit for Modern Life*,
A Toolkit for Happiness and *A Toolkit for Your Emotions*
@psychologymum

Kimberley Wilson
Chartered psychologist and author of *How to Build a Healthy Brain*
@foodandpsych

Lisa Sanfilippo
Psychotherapist, yoga therapist and author of *Sleep Recovery*
www.lisasanfilippo.com

Tim Spector
Professor of genetics and author of *Food for Life* and *Spoon Fed*
@tim.spector

Matthew Syed
Mindset expert and bestselling author of *Rebel Ideas*, *Black Box Thinking* and *Bounce*
matthewsyed.co.uk
@matthewsyedauthor

Daniel G. Amen, MD
Psychiatrist and author of *Change Your Brain Every Day*
daneielamenmd.com
@Doc.Amen

Jay Shetty
Life coach and author of *8 Rules of Love*
@jayshetty

Eckhart Tolle
Spiritual teacher and self-help author of *The Power of Now* and *A New Earth*
EckartTolle.com

Peter Crone
Mind architect
Petercrone.com
@petercrone

Dr Rangan Chatterjee
Podcaster and author of *Happy Mind, Happy Life*, *The Stress Solution* and *The 4 Pillar Plan*
Feel Better Live More podcast
Drchatterjee.com
@drchatterjee

Professor Matthew Walker
Scientist and the director of the Center for Human Sleep Science at the University of California, Berkeley and author of *Why We Sleep*

Brené Brown
Research professor and author of *Daring Greatly*, *Atlas of the Heart* and *The Gifts of Imperfection*
Brenebrown.com
@brenebrown

Pippa Campbell
Female health nutritionist and functional medicine practitioner
Pippacampbellhealth.com
@pippacampbell_health

Mel Robbins
Bestselling author of *The High 5 Habit*
Melrobbins.com
@melrobbins

Dr Alex George
Author of *The Mind Manual*
@dralexgeorge

Dr Angela Holliday-Bell
Sleep specialist
thesolutionissleepcom
@thesleep_md

Dr Gabor Maté
Speaker and author of *When the Body Says No* and
The Myth of Normal
Drgabormate.com
@gabormatemd

Mo Gawdat
Bestselling author of *Solve for Happy* and *Scary Smart*
mogawdat.com
@mo_gowdat

Poppy Jamie
Entrepreneur and author of *Happy Not Perfect*
Happynotperfect.com
@poppyjamie

Megan Rossi
Dietitian, gut health expert and author of *Eat More, Live Well*
Theguthealthdoctor.com
@theguthealthdoctor

Ryan Holiday
Author of *The Daily Stoic, Courage is Calling* and *Discipline is Destiny*
@ryanholiday

Dr Sarah Vohra, aka The Mind Medic
Consultant psychiatrist
themindmedic.co.uk
@themindmedic

Supplements

Bare Biology
barebiology.com
@barebiology

Wild Nutrition
wildnutrition.com
@wildnutritionltd

SuperNova Living
supernovaliving.com
@supernova.living

Naked Pharmacy
thenakedpharmacy.com
@thenakedpharmacy

Form Nutrition
Formnutrition.com
@formnutrition

Artah
Artah.co
@artahhealth

Equi London
equilondon.com
@equilondon

Nutritionists / healthy cooks / movement specialists

Madeleine Shaw
Nutritionist, yoga and meditation teacher
madeleineshaw.com
@madeleine_shaw_

Gem Wade
Home cook
cookwithgem.com
@cookwithgem

Dr Rupy Aujla
NHS medical doctor
thedoctorskitchen.com
@doctors_kitchen

Yumna, Feelgoodfoodie
feelgoodfoodie.net
@Feelgoodfoodie

Dr Libby Weaver
Nutritional biochemist
@drlibby

Deliciously Ella
deliciouslyella.com
@DeliciouslyElla

Emily English
Nutritionist
emilyenglish.com
@Emthenutritionist

James Smith
Personal trainer
@jamesmithpt

Joe Wicks
Fitness coach
thebodycoach.com
@thebodycoach

Roger Frampton
Stretch expert
roger.coach
@rogerframpton

Fiit Fitness App
fiit.tv

Shreddy
shreddy.com
@shreddy

Dr Hazel Wallace
Medical doctor and nutritionist
@thefoodmedic

Isa Welly
Registered nutritional therapist and wellness coach
isawelly.com
@isawelly

Alice Liveing
Personal trainer and author
alice-liveing.co.uk
@aliceliveing

Amelia Freer
Nutritional therapist
ameliafreer.com
@ameliafreer

Melissa Hemsley
Chef
melissahemsley.com
@melissa.hemsley

Frame
Fitness centres
moveyourframe.com
@moveyourframe

Menopause specialists

Dr Louise Newson
GP and renowned menopause specialist
@menopause_doctor

Dr Shahzadi Harper
Menopause specialist and author of *The Perimenopause Solution*
@DrShahzadiharper

Apps

Happy Not Perfect
Headspace
Calm
Insight Timer

Other accounts to follow

Action For Happiness
actionforhappiness.org
@actionforhappiness

Brianna Wiest
Author of *101 Essays That Will Change the Way You Think*
@briannawiest

Helen Marie
Psychotherapy and counselling
helenmarietherapy.com
@h.e.l.e.n.m.a.r.i.e

Wim Hof
Breathwork expert
@iceman_hof
@words_by_wilde_road
@momentaryhappiness

Brands we love

Breathe Lifestyle
breathelifestyle.co.uk

Dirtea
dirteaworld.com

Jones Road
jonesroadbeauty.com

Victoria Health
victoriahealth.com

Ilia
iliabeauty.com

Larq
livelarq.com

One Line A Day journal
www.amazon.co.uk

The Five Minute Journal
intelligentchange.com

Yogi Bare
yogi-bare.co.uk

Aeyla
aeyla.co.uk

Floks
floks.co.uk

NOTES

INTRODUCTION

Page 9   **sleep is the bedrock of better wellbeing:** Amy Gallagher, 'Eight benefits of a good night's sleep', Bupa, 27 October 2021, https://www.bupa.co.uk/newsroom/ourviews/benefits-good-night-sleep

Page 9   **too little sleep has been linked to:** Goran Medic, Micheline Wille and Michael Hemels, 'Short- and long-term health consequences of sleep disruption', *Nature and Science of Sleep*, May 2017, 151–61, https://www.ncbi.nlm.nih.gov/pmc/articles/PMC5449130/

Page 11   **The first is our fight or flight mode:** 'Understanding the stress response', *Harvard Health Publishing*, July 2020, https://www.health.harvard.edu/staying-healthy/understanding-the-stress-response

Page 11   **Stress is vital for two important functions:** Elaine Selna, 'How some stress can actually be good for you', *Time*, November 2018, https://time.com/5434826/stress-good-health/

Page 11   **Studies from the University of California:** Robert Sanders, 'Researchers find out why some stress is good for you', *Berkeley News*, April 2013, https://news.berkeley.edu/2013/

04/16/researchers-find-out-why-some-stress-is-good-for-
you/

Page 12   **Studies from Harvard Medical School:** Toni Golen and
Hope Ricciotti, 'Does exercise really boost energy?', *Harvard
Health Publishing*, July 2021, https://www.health.harvard.
edu/exercise-and-fitness/does-exercise-really-boost-
energy-levels

Page 13   **A recent study from University College London:** 'Middle-
aged adults may be spending more time on the sofa than
previously thought', Centre for Longitudinal Studies, UCL,
October 2020, https://cls.ucl.ac.uk/middle-aged-adults-
may-be-spending-more-time-on-the-sofa-than-
previously-thought/

Page 14   **research into neuroplasticity:** Rick Hanson, 'How to
trick your brain for happiness', *Greater Good Magazine*,
September 2011, https://greatergood.berkeley.edu/article/
item/how_to_trick_your_brain_for_happiness

Page 20   **Plant extracts have been used:** Biljana Bauer Petrovska,
'Historical review of medicinal plants' usage', *Pharma-
cognosy Review* 6(11), January–June 2012, 1–5, https://
www.ncbi.nlm.nih.gov/pmc/articles/PMC3358962/;
Hazem S. Elshafie and Ippolito Camele, 'An overview of
the biological effects of some Mediterranean essential
oils on human health', *Biomed Research International*,
November 2017, https://www.ncbi.nlm.nih.gov/pmc/art-
icles/PMC5694587/

Page 27   **a process called olfaction:** T. Faroqui, 'Olfaction', *Trace
Amines and Neurological Disorders*, 2016, https://www.
sciencedirect.com/topics/neuroscience/olfaction

Page 27   **Different essential oils bring different benefits:** 'Does
aromatherapy using essential oils work?', Consumer
Reports, April 2016, https://www.consumerreports.org/
conditions-treatments/does-aromatherapy-using-
essential-oils-work/

Page 28 **There are some small studies:** 'Dermal absorption of essential oils', *Naturopathic Doctor News & Review* , June 2015, https://ndnr.com/mindbody/dermal-absorption-of-essential-oils/

Page 36 **research shows extreme exercise:** Leigh Weingus and Sheeva Talebian, 'Is your workout messing with your hormones?', MindBodyGreen, October 2019, https://www.mindbodygreen.com/articles/is-your-workout-messing-with-your-hormones

1. SLEEP

Page 43 **spend up to 90 per cent of their day:** 'Daily time spent indoors in German homes – Baseline data for the assessment of indoor exposure of German occupants', *International Journal of Hygiene and Environmental Health* 208(4), July 2005, 247–53, https://www.sciencedirect.com/science/article/abs/pii/S1438463905000635?via%3Dihub

Page 43 **A survey of nearly 17,000 people:** 'Global survey finds we're lacking fresh air and natural light, as we spend less time in nature', Velux Media Centre, May 2019, https//press.velux.com/new-global-survey-finds-were-lacking-fresh-air-and-natural-light-as-we-spend-less-time-in-nature/

Page 43 **what's been called the 'Indoor Generation':** Stephanie Walden, '5 things the "Indoor Generation" can do to be healthier and happier', *USA Today*, https://eu.usatoday.com/story/sponsor-story/velux/2018/05/15/5-things-indoor-generation-can-do-happier-and-healthier/610111002/

Page 44 **circadian rhythm plays a vital role:** 'Circadian rhythms', National Institute of General Medical Sciences, https://nigms.nih.gov/education/fact-sheets/Pages/circadian-rhythms.aspx

Page 44 **getting enough daylight is essential:** 'Sunlight and your health', WebMD, February 2022, https://www.webmd.

com/a-to-z-guides/ss/slideshow-sunlight-health-effects

Page 49 **Well-regulated circadian rhythms:** Danielle Pacheco and Joshua Tal, 'Can you change your circadian rhythm', Sleep Foundation, June 2023, https://www.sleepfoundation.org/circadian-rhythm/can-you-change-your-circadian-rhythm

Page 49 **15 per cent of the UK population:** 'What is shift work?' Indeed, May 2023, https://uk.indeed.com/career-advice/finding-a-job/what-is-shift-work

Page 50 **people who stick to a regular sleep–wake cycle:** Adriane Soehner, Kathy Kennedy and Timothy Monk, 'Circadian preference and saleep-wake regularity: Associations with self-report sleep parameters in daytime-working adults', *Chronobiology International 28*(9), November 2011, 802–9, https://www.tandfonline.com/doi/full/10.3109/07420528.2011.613137

Page 50 **Even losing one hour of sleep:** 'Sleep/wake cycles', Johns Hopkins Medicine, https://www.hopkinsmedicine.org/health/conditions-and-diseases/sleepwake-cycles

Page 50 **Children who have regular bedtimes:** George Kitsaras, Michaela Goodwin, Julia Allan, Michael P. Kelly and Iain A. Pretty, 'Bedtime routines child wellbeing & development', *BMC Public Health*, March 2018, https://www.ncbi.nlm.nih.gov/pmc/articles/PMC5861615/

Page 50 **if we miss out on sleep in the week:** Danielle Pacheco and Dr Anis Rehman, 'Sleep Latency', Sleep Foundation, January 2023, https://www.sleepfoundation.org/how-sleep-works/sleep-latency; Tianyi Huang and Susan Redline, 'Cross-sectional and prospective associations of actigraphy-assessed sleep regularity with metabolic abnormalities: The multi-ethnic study of atheroscleros', *Diabetes Care 42*(8), 2019, 1422–9, https://diabetesjournals.org/care/

article/42/8/1422/36074/Cross-sectional-and-Prospective-Associations-of

Page 51 **'social jet lag' is the specific term:** Rocco Caliandro, Astrid A. Streng, et al., 'Social jetlag and related risks for human health: A timely review', *Nutrients* 13(2), December 2018, https://www.ncbi.nlm.nih.gov/pmc/articles/PMC8707 256/#sec4-nutrients-13-04543title

Page 51 **a Brazilian study on 4,051 adults:** Rocco Caliandro, Astrid A. Streng, et al., 'Social jetlag and related risks for human health: A timely review'

Page 51 **An irregular sleep schedule can affect our metabolism:** 'Study links irregular sleep patterns to metabolic disorder', National Institutes of Health, June 2019, https://www.nih. gov/news-events/news-releases/study-links-irregular-sleep-patterns-metabolic-disorders

Page 51 **Sleep deprivation interferes with our insulin levels:** 'Sleep for a Good Cause', Centers for Disease Control and Prevention, https://www.cdc.gov/diabetes/library/features/diabetes-sleep.html

Page 51 **This makes us 'metabolically groggy':** John Easton, 'Even your fat cells need sleep', University of Chicago News, October 2012, https://news.uchicago.edu/story/even-your-fat-cells-need-sleep-according-new-research

Page 52 **Sleep chronotypes:** Danielle Pacheco and Dr Anis Rehman, 'Chronotypes', Sleep Foundation, July 2023, https://www.sleepfoundation.org/how-sleep-works/chronotypes

Page 53 **Traditionally night owls:** Lynn Marie Trotti, 'Waking up is the hardest thing I do all day: Sleep inertia and sleep drunkenness', *Sleep Medicine Reviews* 35, October 2017, 76–84, https://www.ncbi.nlm.nih.gov/pmc/articles/PMC5337178

Page 54 **government guidelines suggest 7–8 hours:** 'Sleep problems', NHS UK, https://www.nhs.uk/every-mind-matters/mental-health-issues/sleep

Page 54   **we actually sleep in cycles:** Aakash K. Patel, Vamsi Reddy, et al., 'Physiology, sleep stages', StatPearls, September 2022, https://www.ncbi.nlm.nih.gov/books/NBK526132/

Page 54   **Sleep cycles can differ:** 'Sleep physiology', *Sleep Disorders and Sleep Deprivation*, 2006, https://www.ncbi.nlm.nih.gov/books/NBK19956/

Page 55   **Deep sleep is when:** Danielle Pacheco and Dr Abhinav Singh, 'Deep sleep: How much do you need?', Sleep Foundation, July 2023, https://www.sleepfoundation.org/stages-of-sleep/deep-sleep

Page 55   **a 2022 Cambridge University study:** 'Seven hours of sleep is optimal in middle and old age', Cambridge University Press, April 2022, https://www.cam.ac.uk/research/news/seven-hours-of-sleep-is-optimal-in-middle-and-old-age-say-researchers

Page 55   **'deep clean' for the brain:** Kerry Benon, 'Are we "brain washed" during sleep?', The Brink, Boston University, October 2019, https://www.bu.edu/articles/2019/cerebrospinal-fluid-washing-in-brain-during-sleep/

Page 56   **The REM, or rapid eye movement, stage:** 'Learning while you sleep: Dream or reality?', *Harvard Health Publishing*, February 2012, https://www.health.harvard.edu/staying-healthy/learning-while-you-sleep-dream-or-reality

Page 56   **This is the stage where the most vivid dreams happen:** Matthew Walker, 'Why your brain needs to dream', *Greater Good Magazine*, October 2017, https://greatergood.berkeley.edu/article/item/why_your_brain_needs_to_dream

Page 56   **Drinking alcohol decreases REM sleep:** Danielle Pacheco and Dr Abhinav Singh, 'Alcohol and sleep', Sleep Foundation, June 2023, https://www.sleepfoundation.org/nutrition/alcohol-and-sleep

Page 56   **A recent study by the University of Notre Dame:** John Anderer, '5 more minutes! 6 in 10 people habitually hit the snooze button each morning', StudyFinds, October 2018. https://studyfinds.org/hit-the-snooze-button-sleep/

Page 57 **But studies say the opposite:** Stephen M. Mattingly, Gonzalo Martinez, et al., 'Snoozing: An examination of a common method of waking', *Sleep 45*(10), October 2022, https://pubmed.ncbi.nlm.nih.gov/35951011/

Page 57 **every time we hit that snooze button:** Kosuke Kaida, Keiko Ogawa, et al., 'Self-awakening prevents acute rise in blood pressure and heart rate at the time of awakening in elderly people', *Industrial Health 43*(1), 179–85, https://www.jstage.jst.go.jp/article/indhealth/43/1/43_1_179/_article

Page 59 **This is because of something called 'sleep inertia';** Lynn Marie Trotti, 'Waking up is the hardest thing I do all day: Sleep inertia and sleep drunkenness', *Sleep Medicine Reviews 35*, October 2017, 76–84, https://www.ncbi.nlm.nih.gov/pmc/articles/PMC5337178

Page 60 **Morning movement is a great way to wake up:** Cele E. Richardson, Michael Gradisar, Michelle A. Short and Christin Lang, 'Can exercise regulate the circadian system of adolescents? Novel implications for the treatment of delayed sleep-wake phase disorder', *Sleep Medicine Reviews 34*, August 2017, 122–9, https://www.sciencedirect.com/science/article/abs/pii/S1087079216300624?via%3Dihub

Page 60 **even stretching can help wake up the body:** 'Try these stretches before you get out of bed', *Harvard Health Publishing*, April 2010, https://www.health.harvard.edu/staying-healthy/try-these-stretches-before-you-get-out-of-bed; Kate Murray, Suneeta Godbole, et al., 'The relations between sleep, time of physical activity, and time outdoors among adult women', PLOS ONE, September 2017, https://pubmed.ncbi.nlm.nih.gov/28877192/

Page 60 **pink noise could be equally good:** Danielle Pacheco and Dr. Abhinav Singh, 'Can pink noise help you sleep?' Sleep Foundation, January 2023, https://www.sleepfoundation./noise-and-sleep/pink-noise-sleep

Page 60 **journalling can be very cathartic:** Jeremy Sutton, '5 benefits of journaling for mental health', Positive Psychology, May 2018, https://positivepsychology.com/benefits-of-journaling/

Page 62 **Regular light exposure throughout the day:** Katharine A. Kaplan, David C. Talavera and Allison G. Harvey, 'Rise and shine: A treatment experiment testing a morning routine to decrease subjective sleep inertia in insomnia and bipolar disorder', *Behavior Research and Therapy 111*, December 2018, 106–12, https://www.sciencedirect.com/science/article/abs/pii/S0005796718301621

Page 62 **They also play a vital role:** Eric Suni and Kimberley Truong, 'How sleep affects immunity', Sleep Foundation, April 2022, https://www.sleepfoundation.org/physical-health/how-sleep-affects-immunity

Page 62 **linked to people with non-seasonal depression:** Lawrence Epstein and Syed Moin Hassan, 'Why your sleep and wake cycles affect your mood', *Harvard Health Publishing*, May 2020, https://www.health.harvard.edu/blog/why-your-sleep-and-wake-cycles-affect-your-mood-2020051319792#

Page 63 **negative effects of blue light exposure:** 'Blue light has a dark side', *Harvard Health Publishing*, July 2020, https://www.health.harvard.edu/staying-healthy/blue-light-has-a-dark-side

Page 63 **We get natural doses of blue light from the sun:** Rob Newson and Dr Abhinav Singh, 'how blue light affects sleep', Sleep Foundation, March 2023, https://www.sleepfoundation.org/bedroom-environment/blue-light

Page 64 **Light is measured in something called lux:** 'Wake up lights, lux therapy and lux', Wake to Light, November 2015, https://waketolight.com/wake-lights-light-therapy-lux/

Page 66 **A bit about UV light:** 'UVA vs UVB rays: What is the difference?', Paula's Choice Skincare, https://www.paulaschoice.co.uk/the-difference-between-uva-and-uvb-rays

Page 67 **something as simple as sitting by a window:** Mohamed Boubekri et al., 'Impact of windows and daylight exposure on overall health and sleep quality of office workers: A case-control pilot study', *Journal of Clinical Sleep Medicine* 19(6), June 2014, 603–11, https://www.ncbi.nlm.nih.gov/pmc/articles/PMC4031400/

Page 68 **how we move in the day:** Danielle Pacheco and Dr Abhinav Singh, 'Exercise and sleep', Sleep Foundation, March 2023, https://www.sleepfoundation.org/physical-activity/exercise-and-sleep; and Mounir Chennaoui, Pierrick J. Arnal et al., 'Sleep and exercise, a reciprocal issue?', *Sleep Medicine Reviews 20*, April 2015, 59–72, https://www.sciencedirect.com/science/article/abs/pii/S1087079214000720#bib16

Page 68 **New guidelines set in 2020 by the World Health Organization:** 'World Health Organization 2020 guidelines on physical activity and sedentary behaviour', *British Journal of Sports Medicine*, December 2020, 1451–62, https://pubmed.ncbi.nlm.nih.gov/33239350/

Page 68 **Studies show that 30 minutes a day:** 'Benefits of exercise', NHS, https://www.nhs.uk/live-well/exercise/exercise-health-benefits/

Page 72 **it can also lower stress and anxiety:** 'The importance of maintaining structure and routine during stressful times', Very Well Mind, August 2022, https://www.verywellmind.com/the-importance-of-keeping-a-routine-during-stressful-times-4802638

Page 73   **When it comes to alcohol:** 'How long does alcohol stay in
your system?', Healthline, https://www.healthline.com/
health/how-does-alcohol-stay-in-your-system;
Sean He, Brant P. Hasler and Subhajit Chakravorty, 'Alcohol
and sleep related problems', *Current Opinion in Psychology
30*, December 2019, 117–22, https://www.sciencedirect.
com/science/article/pii/S2352250X18302719?via%3Dihub

Page 74   **High activity exercise later in the evening:** 'Does exercising at night affect sleep?', *Harvard Health Publishing*,
April 2019, https://www.health.harvard.edu/staying-
healthy/does-exercising-at-night-affect-sleep

Page 75   **Try doing some gentle stretching:** D. J. Miller, C. Sargent,
et al., 'Moderate-intensity exercise performed in the evening does not impair sleep in healthy males', *European
Journal of Sport Science 20*(1), May 2019, https://www.
tandfonline.com/doi/full/10.1080/17461391.2019.1611934

Page 75   **90 per cent of American adults:** Michael Gradisar, Amy
R. Wolfson, et al., 'The sleep and technology use of Americans: Findings from the National Sleep Foundation's 2011
sleep in America Poll', *Journal of Clinical Sleep Medicine*,
December 2013, 1291–99, https://www.ncbi.nlm.nih.gov/
pmc/articles/PMC3836340/

Page 75   **another good reason we should be putting our screens
down:** Rob Newson and Dr Abhinav Singh, 'How blue
light affects sleep', Sleep Foundation, March 2023, https://
www.sleepfoundation.org/bedroom-environment/
blue-light

Page 75   **A study by Brigham University:** Cami Buckley, 'Is night
shift really helping you sleep better?', BYU News, April
2021, https://news.byu.edu/intellect/is-night-shift-really-
helping-you-sleep-better

Page 76   **Research by the American Academy of Sleep Medicine:**
'New survey: 88% of US adults lose sleep due to binge-
watching', American Academy of Sleep Medicine, September

2019, https://aasm.org/sleep-survey-binge-watching-results/

Page 76 **Binge-watching has also been linked:** Liese Exelmans and Jan Van den Bulck, 'Binge viewing, sleep, and the role of pre-sleep arousal', *Journal of Clinical Sleep Medicine*, August 2017, https://www.ncbi.nlm.nih.gov/pmc/articles/PMC5529125/

Page 78 **gratitude is consistently associated with:** Summer Allen, 'The science of gratitude', The Greater Good Science Center, May 2018, https://ggsc.berkeley.edu/images/uploads/GGSC-JTF_White_Paper-Gratitude-FINAL.pdf

Page 80 **Run a warm bath:** Shahab Haghayegh, Sepideh Khoshnevis, et al., 'Before-bedtime passive body heating by warm shower or bath to improve sleep', *Sleep Medicine Reviews*, August 2019, 124–35, https://www.sciencedirect.com/science/article/abs/pii/S1087079218301552?via%3Dihub

Page 81 **Magnesium is a natural mineral:** Jay Summer and Jenny Iyo, 'How magnesium can help you sleep', Sleep Foundation, July 2023, https://www.sleepfoundation.org/magnesium

Page 81 **increasing our levels improves sleep quality:** Kerri-Ann Jennings, Elizabeth Donovan and Jared Meacham, 'Does magnesium help you sleep better?', Healthline, March 2023, https://www.healthline.com/nutrition/magnesium-and-sleep#what-is-magnesium

Page 82 **Inhalation stimulates the sympathetic system:** Marc A. Russo, Danielle M. Santarelli and Dean O'Rourke, 'The psychological effects of slow breathing in the healthy human', *Breath*, December 2017, 298–309, https://www.ncbi.nlm.nih.gov/pmc/articles/PMC5709795/

Page 83 **we're more likely to interpret other people's facial expressions as hostile:** William D. S. Killgore, Thomas J. Balkin, et al., 'Sleep deprivation impairs recognition of specific emotions', *Neurobiology of Sleep and Circadian*

Rhythms 3, June 2017, 10–16, https://www.sciencedirect.
com/science/article/pii/S2451994416300219?via%3Dihub

Page 84 **four times more likely to catch a cold:** Lisa Marie Potter
and Nicholas Weiler, 'Short sleepers are four times more
likely to catch a cold', University of California San Fran-
cisco, August 2015, https://www.ucsf.edu/news/2015/08/
131411/short-sleepers-are-four-times-more-likely-catch-
cold

Page 84 **affect our consolidation of memories, cognitive performance and our concentration:** 'Memory and Sleep', Sleep
Foundation, April 2023, https://www.sleepfoundation.org/
how-sleep-works/memory-and-sleep

Page 88 **meditation has been shown to slow down the heart rate:**
Daniela Dentico, Fabio Ferrarelli, et al., 'Short meditation
trainings enhance non-REM sleep low-frequency
oscillations', *PLOS ONE*, February 2016, https://pubmed.
ncbi.nlm.nih.gov/26900914/

Page 88 **different types of meditation can help with insomnia:**
Heather L. Rush, Michael Rosario, Lisa M. Levison, et al.,
'The effect of mindfulness meditation on sleep quality: a
systematic review and meta-analysis of randomized controlled trial', *Annals of the New York Academy of Sciences*,
June 2019, 5–16, https://www.ncbi.nlm.nih.gov/pmc/art
icles/PMC6557693/

Page 92 **Most of our lives are spent sitting:** Neville Owen, Phillip
B. Sparling, Geneviève N. Healy, David W. Dunstan and
Charles E. Matthews, 'Sedentary behaviour: Emerging evi-
dence for a new health risk', National library of medicine,
December 2010, https:www.ncbi.nlm.nih.gov/pmc/art
icles/PMC2996155/

Page 95 **participants took longer to fall asleep in a messy bedroom:** Madlen Davies, 'How a MESSY ROOM affects your
sleep: Hoarders take longer to nod off and are more dozy
in the daytime', MailOnline, June 2015, https://www.dai-

lymail.co.uk/health/article-3119867/How-MESSY-ROOM-affects-sleep-Hoarders-longer-nod-dozy-daytime.html

Page 95   **84 per cent of those who'd been working from their bed-room:** Samson Haileyesus, '70% of those working from home experience disrupted sleep patterns', Small Business Trends, July 2020, https://smallbiztrends.com/2020/04/disrupted-sleep-patterns.html

Page 95   **ditching all LED devices (phones, tablets, laptops) before bedtime:** Sarah L. Chellappa, Roland Steiner, Peter Oelhafen, et al., 'Acute exposure to evening blue-enriched light impacts on human sleep', *Journal of Sleep Research*, March 2013, https://onlinelibrary.wiley.com/doi/10.1111/jsr.12050

Page 96   **reading on an iPad suppresses melatonin levels:** Elaine St. Peter, 'E-readers foil good night's sleep', Harvard Medical School, January 2015, https://hms.harvard.edu/news/e-readers-foil-good-nights-sleep

Page 96   **75 per cent of children and 70 per cent of adults use electronic devices:** Eric Suni and Dr Abhinav Singh, 'Technology in the bedroom', Sleep Foundation, December 2022, https://sleepfoundation.org/bedroom-environment/technology-in-the-bedroom

Page 96   **a bedroom that is too warm:** Danielle Pacheco and Heather Wright, 'The best temperature for sleep', Sleep Foundation, July 2023, https://www.sleepfoundation.org/bedroom-environment/best-temperature-for-sleep

Page 97   **evening bath has scientific benefits for sleep:** Nava Zisapek, 'Circadian rhythm sleep disorders', *CNS Drugs*, September 2012,311–28,https://link.springer.com/article/10.2165/00023210-200115040-00005#CR51

Page 97   **having a warm bath activates a process:** Shahab Haghayegh, Sepiden Khoshnevis, et al., 'Before-bedtime passive body heating or bath to improve sleep: A systematic review and meta-analysis', *Sleep Medicine Reviews*,

August 2019, 124–35, https://www.sciencedirect.com/sci-ence/article/abs/pii/S1087079218301552?via%3Dihub

Page 97 **ideal water temperature for an evening soak:** 'Having trouble sleeping? Try a hot bath before bed', Healthline, https://www.healthline.com/health-news/having-trouble-sleeping-try-a-hot-bath-before-bed

Page 97 **Research published in *Sleep Medicine Reviews*:** Shahab Haghayegh, Sepiden Khoshnevis, et al., 'Before-bedtime passive body heating or bath to improve sleep: A system-atic review and meta-analysis'

Page 97 **80 per cent of the world lives under light-polluted skies:** Ben Panko, 'Nighttime light pollution covers nearly 80% of the globe', *Science*, June 2016, https://www.science.org/content/article/nighttime-light-pollution-covers-nearly-80-globe

Page 98 **help with things like stress reduction and anxiety:** 'Anx-iety and stress weighing heavily at night? A new blanket might help', *Harvard Health Publishing*, March 2019, https://www.health.harvard.edu/mind-and-mood/anxiety-and-stress-weighing-heavily-at-night-a-new-blanket-might-help

Page 98 **Sticking to regular mealtimes throughout the day:** 'How eating feeds into the body clock', *Science Daily*, April 2019, https://www.sciencedaily.com/releases/2019/04/190425 143607.htm

Page 99 **we should be basing our days around our mealtimes:** Marie-Pierre St-Onge, Anja Mikic and Cara E. Pietrolungo, 'Effects of diet on sleep quality', *Advances in Nutrition*, September 2016, 938–49, https://www.ncbi.nlm.nih.gov/pmc/articles/PMC5015038/

Page 99 **the cells in our body are primed to follow their own nat-ural daily rhythms:** Ueli Schibler, 'The daily rhythms of genes, cells and organs', *EMBO Reports* 6(1), July 2005, https://www.ncbi.nlm.nih.gov/pmc/articles/PMC1369272/

Page 106 **there are proven scientific benefits to caffeine:** 'Caffeine', Harvard T. H. Chan School of Public Health, https://www.hsph.harvard.edu/nutritionsource/caffeine/; 'Caffeinated or not, coffee linked with longer life', Harvard T.H. Chan, School of Public Health, https://www.hsph.harvard.edu/news/hsph-in-the-news/coffee-longer-life/

Page 107 **it has a half-life of 5–6 hours:** Kristeen Cherney, 'How long does caffeine stay in your system?', Healthline, November 2018, https://www.healthline.com/health/how-long-does-caffeine-last

Page 108 **caffeine doesn't actually give us a buzz:** 'Tired or wired? Caffeine and your brain', News in Health, October 2020, https://newsinhealth.nih.gov/2020/10/tired-or-wired

2. STRESS

Page 113 **YouGov revealed that 74 per cent of respondents:** 'Stressed nation: 74% of UK "overwhelmed or unable to cope" at some point in the past year', Mental Health Foundation, May 2018, https://www.mentalhealth.org.uk/about-us/news/survey-stressed-nation-UK-overwhelmed-unable-to-cope#

Page 118 **statistics show that women suffer more with stress:** Josie Cox, 'Why women are more burned out than men', BBC Worklife, October 2021, https://www.bbc.com/worklife/article/20210928-why-women-are-more-burned-out-than-men

Page 118 **with women making up approximately 80 per cent of diagnosed cases:** Fariha Angum, Tahir Khan, et al., 'The prevalence of autoimmune disorders in women: A narrative review', Cureus, May 2020, https://www.ncbi.nlm.nih.gov/pmc/articles/PMC7292717/#:~:text=There%20are%20over%20100%20types,diseases%20are%20women%20%5B1%5D.

Page 120 **exercise and movement helps to reduce:** 'Exercising to relax', *Harvard Health Publishing*, July 2020, https://www.health.harvard.edu/staying-healthy/exercising-to-relax

Page 121 **altruistic behaviour releases endorphins in the brain:** Jeanie Lerche Davis, 'The science of good deeds', Health & Balance, WebMD, https://www.webmd.com/balance/features/science-good-deeds#:~:text=Altruistic%20behavior%20may%20also%20trigger,body%20naturally%20produces%2C%20Fricchione%20explains.

Page 122 **studies show that engaging in a creative pursuit:** Ashley Stahl, 'Here's how creativity actually helps your health', *Forbes*, July 2018, https://www.forbes.com/sites/ashley-stahl/2018/07/25/heres-how-creativity-actually-improves-your-health/?sh=1e335a2113a6

Page 124 **it can help you get control over your body and brain:** Rebecca Joy Stanborough, 'What to know about cold water therapy', Healthline, March 2023, https://www.healthline.com/health/cold-water-therapy#benefits

Page 125 **Interaction with animals has been shown:** 'The power of pets', News in Health, February 2018, https://newsinhealth.nih.gov/2018/02/power-pets#:~:text=Interacting%20with%20animals%20has%20been,support%2C%20and%20boost%20your%20mood

Page 135 **95 per cent of serotonin production:** Natalie Terry and Kara Gross Margolis, 'Serotonergic mechanisms regulating the GI tract: Experimental evidence and therapeutic relevance', *Handbook of Experimental Pharmacology*, July 2017, 319–42, https://www.ncbi.nlm.nih.gov/pmc/articles/PMC5526216/

Page 135 **The gut also plays a key role:** Dominik W. Schmid, Pablo Capilla-Lashera, et al., 'Circadian rhythms of hosts and their gut microbiomes: Implications for animal physiology and ecology', *Functional Ecology*, January 2023, https://besjournals.onlinelibrary.wiley.com/doi/10.1111/1365-2435.14255

Page 135   **plays an important part in hormonal health:** Brandilyn A. Peters, Nanette Santoro, Robert C. Kaplan and Qibin Qi, 'Spotlight on the gut microbiome in menopause: Current insights', *International Journal of Women's Health*, August 2022, 1059–72, https://www.ncbi.nlm.nih.gov/pmc/articles/PMC9379122/

Page 135   **one of the biggest influences on our gut health:** Annelise Madison and Janice K. Kiecolt-Glaser, 'Stress, depression, diet, and the gut microbiota: Human–bacteria interactions at the core of psychoneuroimmunology and nutrition', *Current Opinion in Behavioral Sciences*, August 2019, 105–10, https://www.ncbi.nlm.nih.gov/pmc/articles/PMC7213601/#:~:text=Additionally%2C%20stress%20and%20depression%20can,alter%20eating%20behavior%20and%20mood

Page 135   **The gut–brain axis is the signalling system:** Dr Sanil Rege and Dr James Graham, 'The simplified guide to the gut-brain axis: How the gut and brain talk to each other', Psych Scene Hub, June 2017, https://psychscenehub.com/psychinsights/the-simplified-guide-to-the-gut-brain-axis/

Page 136   **referred to as the 'information superhighway':** Katherine Gould, 'The vagus nerve: Your body's communication superhighway', LiveScience, September 2022, https://www.livescience.com/vagus-nerve.html

Page 136   **something called vagal tone:** 'Vagus nerve stimulation', Wim Hof Method, https://www.wimhofmethod.com/vagus-nerve-stimulation

Page 136   **Healthy vagal tone means better emotional regulation:** Katie A. McLaughlin, Leslie Rith-Najarian, et al., 'Low vagal tone magnifies the association between psychosocial stress exposure and internalizing psychopathology in adolescents', *Journal of Clinical Child & Adolescent Psychology*, October 2013, https://www.ncbi.nlm.nih.gov/pmc/articles/PMC4076387/

Page 137   **Poor microbiome health has also been linked:** Boshen
Gong, Chuyuan Wang, Fanrui Meng, et al., 'Association
between gut microbiota and autoimmune thyroid disease: A systematic review and meta-analysis', *Frontiers in
Endocrinology*, November 2021, https://www.ncbi.nlm.
nih.gov/pmc/articles/PMC8635774/

Page 137   **people with major depressive disorders may often lack
certain microbes:** Miguel A. Ortega, Miguel Angel Alvarez-
Mon, et al., 'Gut microbiota metabolites in major depressive
disorder—deep insights into their pathophysiological role
and potential translational applications', *Metabolites*,
January 2022, https://www.ncbi.nlm.nih.gov/pmc/art-
icles/PMC8778125/

Page 139   **recent research from the American Gut Project:** 'Big data
from the world's largest citizen science microbiome project
serves food for thought', *Science Daily*, May 2018, https://
www.sciencedaily.com/releases/2018/05/180515092931.htm

Page 140   **Probiotics are essentially live beneficial bacteria:** 'Probiotics: What you need to know', National Center for
Complementary and Integrative Health, https://www.
nccih.nih.gov/health/probiotics-what-you-need-to-know

Page 142   **there is a link between sugar and stress:** Sara Lindberg
and Erin Kelly, 'Your anxiety loves sugar: Eat these 3 things
instead', Healthline, June 2020, https://www.healthline.
com/health/mental-health/how-sugar-harms-mental-
health#worsen-anxiety

Page 143   **Some studies suggest that willpower:** Nir Eyal, 'Have we
been thinking about willpower the wrong way for 30 years?'
Harvard Business Review, November 2016, https://hbr.
org/2016/11/have-we-been-thinking-about-willpower-
the-wrong-way-for-30-years; Jeremy Sutton, 'What is
willpower? The psychology behind self-control', Positive
Psychology, October 2016, https://positivepsychology.
com/psychology-of-willpower/

Page 145 **The power of nature on our wellbeing is backed by science:** Jim Robbins, 'Ecopsychology: How immersion in nature benefits your health', Yale Environment 360, January 2020, https://e360.yale.edu/features/ecopsychology-how-immersion-in-nature-benefits-your-health#:~:text= These%20studies%20have%20shown%20that,reduce%20 anxiety%2C%20and%20improve%20mood; 'A 20-minute nature break relieves stress', *Harvard Health Publishing*, July 2019, https://www.health.harvard.edu/mind-and-mood/ a-20-minute-nature-break-relieves-stress

Page 145 **A University of Sussex study found:** 'It's true – the sound of nature helps us relax', Brighton and Sussex Medical School, 2017, https://www.bsms.ac.uk/about/news/2017/ 03-31-the-sound-of-nature-helps-us-relax.aspx

Page 146 **A 2021 US review:** Rachel T. Buxton, Amber L. Pearson, Claudia Allou and George Wittemyer, 'A synthesis of health benefits of natural sounds and their distribution in national parks', *The Proceedings of the National Academy of Sciences 118*(14), March 2021, https://www.pnas.org/ doi/10.1073/pnas.2013097118

Page 146 **Studies measuring the levels of cortisol:** Alan Ewert and Yun Chang, 'Levels of nature and stress response', *Behavioral Sciences (Basel)*, May 2018, https://www.ncbi.nlm. nih.gov/pmc/articles/PMC5981243/

Page 146 **A study of 20,000 people by Exeter University:** Prof. Ruth Garside, 'Attention restoration theory: A systematic review', European Centre for Environment & Human Health, University of Exeter Medical School, https://www.ecehh.org/ research/attention-restoration-theory-a-systematic-review/#:~:text=Background,in%20'directed%20 attention%20fatigue'

Page 147 **A joint UK and New Zealand study:** Ben Gooden, 'A green view: How seeing trees from your window improves wellbeing', Citygreen, June 2019, https://citygreen.com/

a-green-view-how-seeing-trees-from-your-window-
improves-wellbeing/

Page 154 **proven benefits for reducing stress:** Emma Seppälä,
Christina Bradley and Michael R. Goldstein, 'Research:
Why breathing is so effective for stress', *Harvard Business
Review*, September 2020, https://hbr.org/2020/09/research-
why-breathing-is-so-effective-at-reducing-stress

3. ENERGY

Page 161 **'tired all the time', according to the NHS:** Isabelle Kirk,
'One in eight Britons feel tired all the time', YouGov, January
2022, https://yougov.co.uk/topics/society/articles-reports/
2022/01/11/one-eight-britons-feel-tired-all-time

Page 161 **Three in five Americans say:** 'Exhausted nation: Americans more tired than ever, survey finds', *Family Safety &
Health*, January 2022, https://www.safetyandhealthmaga-
zine.com/articles/22112-exhausted-nation-americans-
more-tired-than-ever-survey-finds

Page 162 **a quarter of adults felt tired:** Isabelle Kirk, 'One in eight
Britons feel tired all the time', YouGov, January 2022,
https://yougov.co.uk/topics/society/articles-reports/
2022/01/11/one-eight-britons-feel-tired-all-time

Page 162 **A 2021 YouGov survey on families:** 'Families and the
labour market, UK: 2021', YouGov, July 2022, https://www.
ons.gov.uk/employmentandlabourmarket/peopleinwork/
employmentandemployeetypes/articles/familiesandthe-
labourmarketengland/2021#:~:text=In%20March%20
2022%2C%20employed%20women,minutes%20per%20
day%2C%20respectively

Page 162 **Survey from marketing research company**: 'Energy
crisis: 3 in 5 Americans move exhausted now than ever in
their lives', Studyfinds, https://studyfinds.org/exhausted-
nation-pandemic-tired-energy

Page 165 **dehydrated by just 2 per cent impairs:** Ana Adan, 'Cognitive performance and dehydration', *Journal of the American College of Nutrition*, April 2012, https://pubmed.ncbi.nlm.nih.gov/22855911/

Page 170 **even the gentlest of movement:** Toni Golen and Hope Ricciotti, 'Does exercise really boost energy levels?', *Harvard Health Publishing*, July 2021, https://www.health.harvard.edu/exercise-and-fitness/does-exercise-really-boost-energy-levels

Page 170 **Journalling has been proven to help:** Jeremy Sutton, '5 benefits of journaling for mental health', Positive Psychology, May 2018, https://positivepsychology.com/benefits-of-journaling/

Page 170 **Drink your coffee between 9.30am and 11.30am:** 'When is the best time to drink coffee?', Healthline, https://www.healthline.com/nutrition/best-time-to-drink-coffee#cortisol-coffee

Page 171 **listening to our favourite music:** Eric W. Dolan, 'Listening to the music you love will make your brain release more dopamine, study finds', PsyPost, February 2019, https://www.psypost.org/2019/02/listening-to-the-music-you-love-will-make-your-brain-release-more-dopamine-study-finds-53059

Page 171 **Turn the shower to cold for 30 seconds:** Geert A. Buijze, Inger N. Sierevelt, et al., 'The effect of cold showering on health and work: A randomized controlled trial', *PLoS One*, September 2015, https://www.ncbi.nlm.nih.gov/pmc/articles/PMC5025014/; Lindsay Bottoms, 'Cold showers boost immune systems and increase energy levels, study shows', World Economic Forum, April 2022, https://www.weforum.org/agenda/2022/04/cold-shower-ice-bath-health-wellbeing/

Page 172 **Being outside in nature makes people feel more alive:** University of Rochester, 'Spending time in nature makes

people feel more alive, study shows', *Science Daily*, June
2010, https://www.sciencedaily.com/releases/2010/06/100
603172219.htm

Page 173 **ward off feelings of exhaustion:** Alan Ewert and Yun
Chang, 'Levels of nature and stress response', *Behavioral
Sciences (Basel)*, May 2018, https://www.ncbi.nlm.nih.
gov/pmc/articles/PMC5981243/

Page 173 **children who have green spaces:** Kirsten Weir, 'Nurtured
by nature', *Monitor on Psychology*, American Psychological Association, April 2020, https://www.apa.org/
monitor/2020/04/nurtured-nature

Page 173 **One Australian study gave participants:** Nicole Torres,
'Gazing at nature makes you more productive', *Harvard
Business Review*, September 2015, https://hbr.org/2015/09/
gazing-at-nature-makes-you-more-productive

Page 175 **Stretching increases the circulation:** Daniel Yetman, 'The
benefits of stretching and why it feels good', Healthline,
August 2020, https://www.healthline.com/health/why-
does-stretching-feel-good

Page 176 **reduce the meeting time by 25 per cent:** Neal Taparia,
'Kick The Chair: How standing cut our meeting times
by 25%', *Forbes*, June 2014, https://www.forbes.com/
sites/groupthink/2014/06/19/kick-the-chair-how-stand
ing-cut-our-meeting-times-by-25/?sh=e2c307035fed

Page 176 **known for their aromatherapeutic benefits:** Eriko Kawai,
Ryosuke Takeda, et al., 'Increase in diastolic blood pressure
induced by fragrance inhalation of grapefruit essential
oil is positively correlated with muscle sympathetic
nerve activity', *The Journal of Physiological Sciences*,
January 2020, https://www.ncbi.nlm.nih.gov/pmc/articles/
PMC6992548/; Katrina Weston-Green, Helen Clunas and
Carlos Jimenez Naranjo, 'A review of the potential use of
pinene and linalool as terpene-based medicines for brain
health: Discovering novel therapeutics in the flavours and

NOTES

fragrances of cannabis', *Frontiers in Psychiatry*, August 2021, https://www.ncbi.nlm.nih.gov/pmc/articles/PMC8426550/; Pooja Agarwal, Zahra Sebghatollahi, et al., 'Citrus essential oils in aromatherapy: Therapeutic effects and mechanisms', *Antioxidants* (*Basel*), November 2022, https://www.ncbi.nlm.nih.gov/pmc/articles/PMC9774566/

Page 178 **A study published in *Nature Medicine*:** Emmanuel Stamatakis, Matthew N. Ahmadi, et al., 'Association of wearable device-measured vigorous intermittent lifestyle physical activity with mortality', *Nature Medicine*, December 2022, https://www.nature.com/articles/s41591-022-02100-x; Sarah Berry, 'Carrying the shopping bags and walking quickly up stairs helps you live longer', *The Sydney Morning Herald*, December 2022, https://www.smh.com.au/lifestyle/health-and-wellness/carrying-the-shopping-bags-and-walking-quickly-up-stairs-helps-you-live-longer-20221208-p5c4oj.html

Page 179 **research shows that anything between 5,000 and 8,000 steps:** I-Min Lee, Eric J. Shiroma, et al., 'Association of step volume and intensity with all-cause mortality in older women', *JAMA Internal Medicine*, August 2019, https://pubmed.ncbi.nlm.nih.gov/31141585/

Page 179 **study published in the *Journal of Strength and Conditioning*:** David C. Hughes, Stian Ellefsen and Keith Baar, 'Adaptations to endurance and strength training', *Cold Spring Harbor Perspectives in Medicine*, June 2018, https://www.ncbi.nlm.nih.gov/pmc/articles/PMC5983157/

Page 180 **One study published in the journal *PLOS One*:** Muhammad Mustafa Atakan, Yanchun Li, et al., 'Evidence-based effects of high-intensity interval training on exercise capacity and health: A review with historical perspective', *International Journal of Environmental Research and Public Health*, July 2021, https://www.ncbi.nlm.nih.gov/pmc/articles/PMC8294064/

279

Page 180 **5 minutes of stair climbing per day:** Emily C. Dunford, Sydney E. Valentino, Jonathan Dubberley, et al., 'Brief vigorous stair climbing effectively improves cardiorespiratory fitness in patients with coronary artery disease: A randomized trial', *Frontiers in Sports and Active Living*, February 2021, https://www.ncbi.nlm.nih.gov/pmc/articles/PMC7921461/

Page 183 **It's important for our long-term energy:** Meg Walters, 'How does protein give you energy?', Live Science, July 2022, https://www.livescience.com/how-does-protein-give-you-energy

Page 184 **supporting brain health:** 'Could intermittent fasting help maintain a healthy brain?', Zoe, August 2023, https://join-zoe.com/learn/intermittent-fasting-and-brain-health

Page 188 **consuming two to three cups of coffee a day:** Nina Massey, 'Drinking two to three cups of coffee a day linked with longer lifespan, study finds', *Independent*, September 2022, https://www.independent.co.uk/news/health/coffee-caffeine-cups-longer-life-b2176119

Page 188 **Coffee contains up to 100 biologically active ingredients:** James H. O'Keefe, James J. DiNicolantonio and Carl J. Lavie, 'Coffee for cardioprotection and longevity', *Progress in Cardiovascular Diseases*, May–June 2018, https://pubmed.ncbi.nlm.nih.gov/29474816/

Page 188 **benefits that support the heart:** Sophia Antipolis, 'Coffee drinking is associated with increased longevity', European Society of Cardiology, September 2022, https://www.escardio.org/The-ESC/Press-Office/Press-releases/Coffee-drinking-is-associated-with-increased-longevity

Page 188 **Studies show that Lion's Mane mushroom:** Erica Julson, '9 health benefits of lion's mane mushroom (Plus Side Effects), Healthline, June 2023, https://www.healthline.com/nutrition/lions-mane-mushroom#reduces-heart-disease-risk

Page 189 **Our resting metabolic rate can go up:** Scott Frothingham, 'What is basal metabolic rate?', Healthline, May 2023, https://www.healthline.com/health/what-is-basal-metabolic-rate

Page 191 **measures of optimism had higher levels:** Suzanne C. Segerstrom, 'Optimism and immunity: Do positive thoughts always lead to positive effects?', *Brain, Behavior, and Immunity*, May 2005, 195–200, https://www.sciencedirect.com/science/article/abs/pii/S0889159104001205

Page 192 **a person's emotional state can impact:** Sanne M. A. Lamers, Linda Bolier, et al., 'The impact of emotional well-being on long-term recovery and survival in physical illness: A meta-analysis', *Journal of Behavioral Medicine*, September 2011, https://www.ncbi.nlm.nih.gov/pmc/articles/PMC3439612/

Page 195 **Fruits, vegetables and grains are a lot less nutritious:** Stacey Colino, 'Fruits and vegetables are less nutritious than they used to be', *National Geographic*, May 2022, https://www.nationalgeographic.co.uk/environment-and-conservation/2022/05/fruits-and-vegetables-are-less-nutritious-than-they-used-to-be

Page 197 **magnesium plays many crucial roles:** Megan Ware, 'Why do we need magnesium?', *Medical News Today*, March 2023, https://www.medicalnewstoday.com/articles/286839

Page 197 **large numbers of us don't get enough magnesium:** Sara Karlovitch, 'Half of all Americans are magnesium deficient', *Pharmacy Times*, July 2020, https://www.pharmacytimes.com/view/study-half-of-all-americans-are-magnesium-deficient

Page 201 **a person uses up 320 calories:** 'Does thinking burn calories? Here's what the science says', *Time*, September 2018, https://time.com/5400025/does-thinking-burn-calories

4. MOOD

Page 205 **we have a lot more agency over our happiness:** Kira M. Newman, 'How much of your happiness is under your control?' *Greater Good Magazine*, February 2020, https://greatergood.berkeley.edu/article/item/how_much_of_your_happiness_is_under_your_control

Page 205 **Happiness can be a spectrum:** Courtney E. Ackerman, 'What is happiness and why is it important?', Positive Psychology, February 2019, https://positivepsychology.com/what-is-happiness/

Page 209 **Values are a really important piece:** Tchiki David, 'Happiness values', Berkeley Well-Being Institute, https://www.berkeleywellbeing.com/happiness-values-activity.html

Page 211 **Neuroplasticity is a hot topic:** Eagle Gamma, 'Brain plasticity (neuroplasticity): How experience changes the brain', *Simply Psychology*, July 2023, https://www.simplypsychology.org/brain-plasticity.html

Page 212 **Epigenetics is another emerging area:** 'What is epigenetics?' Centers for Disease Control and Prevention, https://www.cdc.gov/genomics/disease/epigenetics.htm

Page 213 **Positive psychology is a relatively new branch:** 'Positive psychology', *Harvard Health Publishing*, https://www.health.harvard.edu/topics/positive-psychology

Page 214 **Research has found that a daily writing practice:** Joshua M. Smyth, Jillian A. Johnson, Brandon J. Auer, et al., 'Online positive affect journaling in the improvement of mental distress and well-being in general medical patients with elevated anxiety symptoms: A preliminary randomized controlled trial', *JMIR Mental Health*, October–December 2018, https://www.ncbi.nlm.nih.gov/pmc/articles/PMC6305886/

Page 214 **showed a 28 per cent reduction in stress levels:** 'Gratitude is good medicine', UC Davis Health, November 2015,

https://health.ucdavis.edu/medicalcenter/features/2015-
2016/11/20151125_gratitude.html

Page 214 **asked participants to write:** 'Writing a thank you note is
more powerful than you think', *Harvard Health Publishing*,
February 2021, https://www.health.harvard.edu/mind-and-
mood/writing-a-thank-you-note-is-more-powerful-
than-you-think

Page 216 **Hope theory:** C. R. Snyder, Keven L. Rand and David
R. Sigmon, 'Hope theory', https://teachingpsychology.
files.wordpress.com/2012/02/hope-theory.pdf

Page 218 **A growth mindset is the belief:** Sarah D. Sparks, '"Growth
mindset" linked to higher test scores, student well-being
in global study', *Education Week*, April 2021, https://www.
edweek.org/leadership/growth-mindset-linked-to-
higher-test-scores-student-well-being-in-global-
study/2021/04

Page 219 **People are generally happier with their lives:** Dr Louis Tay,
'The amazing benefits of happiness', Purdue University,
March 2021, https://www.purdue.edu/stepstoleaps/explore/
well-being-tips/well-being-tips-2021/2021_0308.php#

Page 220 **the Happiness Research Institute found:** Zach Johnson,
'How brands can deliver unique, memorable experiences
in customers' everyday lives', Marketing Week, https://
www.marketingweek.com/brands-unique-memorable-
experiences-customers-everyday-lives/

Page 220 **The 'Flow' state is a term coined:** Mike Oppland, '8 traits
of flow according to Mihaly Csikszentmihalyi', Positive
Psychology, December 2016, https://positivepsychology.
com/mihaly-csikszentmihalyi-father-of-flow/#

Page 222 **'ordinary magic':** A. S. Masten, 'Ordinary magic: Resilience
processes in development', *American Psychologist 56*(3),
227–38, https://psycnet.apa.org/record/2001-00465-004

Page 225 **performing small acts of kindness:** 'The science of kindness', Random Acts of Kindness Foundation, https://www.randomactsofkindness.org/the-science-of-kindness

Page 225 **a 2013 study found a link between volunteering:** '7 scientific facts about the benefit of doing good', Goodnet, January2017,https://www.goodnet.org/articles/7-scientific-facts-about-benefit-doing-good

Page 225 **the science of giving:** 'Giving thanks can make you happier', *Harvard Health Publishing*, August 2021, https://www.health.harvard.edu/healthbeat/giving-thanks-can-make-you-happier

Page 225 **Leading happiness researcher Sonja Lyubomirsky:** Megan M. Fritz and Sonja Lyubomirsky, 'Whither happiness?' https://sonjalyubomirsky.com/files/2012/09/Fritz-Lyubomirsky-in-press-1.pdf

Page 226 **studies consistently show that sleep deprivation:** 'Sleep and mood', Division of Sleep Medicine, Harvard Medical School, https://sleep.hms.harvard.edu/education-training/public-education/sleep-and-health-education-program/sleep-health-education-87; Kimberley Holland, 'Why a lack of sleep can make you angry', Healthline, December 2018, https://www.healthline.com/health-news/why-a-lack-of-sleep-can-make-you-angry

Page 226 **2019 Iowa State University study:** 'Lack of sleep intensifies anger, impairs adaptation to frustrating circumstances', Iowa State University, November 2018, https://www.news.iastate.edu/news/2018/11/27/sleepanger

Page 226 **average amount of sleep a person needs:** Scott Frothingham, 'Is 5 hours enough sleep?' Healthline, May 2019, https://www.healthline.com/health/is-5-hours-enough-sleep

Page 226 **we also tend to eat less healthily:** Eric Suni and John DeBanto, 'Sleep and overeating', Sleep Foundation, April 2022, https://www.sleepfoundation.org/physical-health/sleep-and-overeating#references-82712

Page 227 **we're more likely to reach for calorie-dense:** Stephanie M. Greer, Andrea M. Goldstein and Matthew P. Walker, 'The impact of sleep deprivation on food desire in the human brain', *Nature Communications*, 2013, https://pubmed. ncbi.nlm.nih.gov/23922121/

Page 227 **Omega 3 is essential for:** James J. DiNicolantonio and James H. O'Keefe, 'The importance of marine omega-3s for brain development and the prevention and treatment of behavior, mood, and other brain disorders', *Nutrients*, August 2020, https://www.ncbi.nlm.nih.gov/pmc/articles/PMC7468918/

Page 227 **Don't forget the B vitamins:** Duaa Durrani, Rahma Idrees, Hiba Idrees and Aayat Ellahi, 'Vitamin B6: A new approach to lowering anxiety, and depression?', *Annals of Medicine & Surgery*, October 2022, https://www.ncbi.nlm.nih.gov/ pmc/articles/PMC9577631/

Page 228 **An influential US study:** James H. Fowler and Nicholas A. Christakis, 'Dynamic spread of happiness in a large social network: Longitudinal analysis over 20 years in the Framingham Heart Study', *British Medical Journal*, September 2008, https://www.bmj.com/content/337/bmj.a2338

Page 228 **happiness can belong to a larger group of people:** Eshin Jolly, Diana I. Tamir, et al., 'Wanting without enjoying: The social value of sharing experience', *Plos One*, April 2019, https://www.ncbi.nlm.nih.gov/pmc/articles/PMC6472755/

Page 228 **respondents matched their mood:** Christine Yu, 'Misery really does love company. Here's how to avoid catching bad moods', Headspace, https://www.headspace.com/art-icles/catching-bad-moods

Page 229 **rude people tend to cluster in groups:** Laura Petitta, Tahira M. Probst, Valerio Ghezzi and Claudio Barbaranelli, 'The impact of emotional contagion on workplace safety: Investigating the roles of sleep, health, and production pressure', *Current Psychology*, March 2021, https://www. ncbi.nlm.nih.gov/pmc/articles/PMC7972334/

Page 229 **A 2022 Bath University study:** 'Social media break improves mental health – new study', Bath University, May 2022, https://www.bath.ac.uk/announcements/social-media-break-improves-mental-health-new-study/

Page 230 **2021 Ofcom survey:** Catherine Hily, 'UK mobile phone statistics, 2023', U Switch, February 2023, https://www.uswitch.com/mobiles/studies/mobile-statistics/#:~:text=Accord ing%20to%20a%202021%20Ofcom,those%20aged%2035%20and%20under.

Page 230 **TikTok was the fastest growing news source:** 'Instagram, TikTok and YouTube teenagers' top three news sources', Ofcom, July 2022, https://www.ofcom.org.uk/news-centre/2022/instagram,-tiktok-and-youtube-teenagers-top-three-news-sources

Page 230 **global survey looking at social media:** Amy Watson, 'Share of adults who use social media as a source of news in selected countries worldwide as of February 2023', Statista, https://www.statista.com/statistics/718019/social-media-news-source/

Page 230 **access the networks on a daily basis:** Andrew Hutchinson, 'New research shows that 71% of Americans now get news content via social platforms', Social Media Today, January 2021, https://www.socialmediatoday.com/news/new-research-shows-that-71-of-americans-now-get-news-content-via-social-pl/593255/

Page 230 **negative news made up 85 per cent:** 'UK tops the charts for negative news stories', PRmoment.com, June 2019, https://www.prmoment.com/pr-research/uk-tops-the-charts-for-negative-news-stories#:~:text=At%20a%20total%20level%20from,positive%2015%25%20of%20the%20time.

Page 230 **'Doomscrolling':** Jessica Klein, 'Why does endlessly looking for bad news feel so strangely gratifying – and can we break the habit?', BBC Worklife, March 2021, https://www.bbc.com/worklife/article/20210226-the-darkly-soothing-compulsion-of-doomscrolling#:~:text= Most%20of%20us%20spent%20some,really%20a%20 new%20human%20behaviour.

Page 231 **A study published in the *British Journal of Psychology*:** Wendy M. Johnston and Graham C. L. Davey, 'The psychological impact of negative TV news bulletins: The catastrophizing of personal worries', *British Journal of Psychology*, April 2011, https://bpspsychub.onlinelibrary. wiley.com/doi/abs/10.1111/j.2044-8295.1997.tb02622.x

Page 231 **a survey of 1,000 people:** Joe Berry, 'How long do Brits spend on their phones?', Lenstore.co.uk, January 2022, https://blog.int.lenstore.co.uk/how-long-do-brits-spend-on-their-phones/

Page 232 **the mood boosting benefits of being out in nature:** Kirsten Weir, 'Nurtured by nature', American Psychological Association, April 2020, https://www.apa.org/ monitor/2020/04/nurtured-nature

Page 232 **Nature can induce in us a sense of awe:** Carolyn Gregoire, 'How awe-inspiring experiences can make you happier, less stressed and more creative', *Huffington Post*, December 2017, https://www.huffingtonpost.co.uk/ entry/the-psychology-of-awe_n_5799850

Page 234 **Biophilic office design:** 'Biophilic office design: The science, benefits and examples', Knight Frank, https://www. knightfrank.co.uk/office-space/insights/culture-and-space/biophilic-office-design/

Page 234 **the social benefits of shared exercise:** Kevin C. Young, Kyla A. Machell, Todd B. Kashdan and Margaret L. Westwater, 'The cascade of positive events: Does exercise on a given day increase the frequency of additional positive events?', *Personality and Individual Differences*, January 2018, https://www.sciencedirect.com/science/article/abs/ pii/S0191886917302027

Page 235 **brief, low-intensity episodes of physical:** Kevin C. Young, Kyla A. Machell, Todd B. Kashdan and Margaret L. Westwater, 'The cascade of positive events: Does exercise on a given day increase the frequency of additional positive events?', *Personality and Individual Differences*, January 2018, https://www.sciencedirect.com/science/article/abs/pii/S0191886917302027